"As a health anxiety specialist, I applaud K[illegible]s understand that the illness they fear is not [illegible]y about fatal diseases, *Freedom from Health Anxiety* is a must-read. Cassiday provides real-life examples, captures the torturous inner dialogue of people who suffer needlessly, and then provides a way out with exercises and tools."

—**Ken Goodman, LCSW**, board member of the Anxiety and Depression Association of America (ADAA), and creator of *The Anxiety Solution Series*

"Karen Lynn Cassiday is one of the leading experts in the anxiety field, not only because she is knowledgeable, but because she has a way of translating information for health anxiety sufferers to understand and use immediately in their lives. *Freedom from Health Anxiety* is packed with success stories, specific strategies, and meaningful ways to change how you respond to your health worries. This book is exactly what you need to take back your life from health anxiety!"

—**Kimberly Morrow, LCSW**, anxiety therapist, author, national speaker, and co-owner of www.anxietytraining.com

"Karen Cassiday compassionately outlines a clear blueprint for dealing with anxiety about illness, dying, and death. Read this wonderful book to learn from a master clinician how to live a happy life even with medical uncertainty."

—**Elizabeth DuPont Spencer, LCSW-C**, co-owner of Anxiety Training

"Karen Cassiday has written a helpful book on how to incorporate creative exposure and response prevention (ERP) exercises into the treatment of health anxiety. The guidance offered throughout is straightforward and easy to implement. Readers will learn how to use gratitude to counterbalance the negative chatter that anxiety injects into one's unfolding experience. I will be recommending this book to my clients looking for additional support working on moving past health anxiety."

—**Debra Kissen, PhD, MHSA**, CEO of Light on Anxiety, author of *Rewire Your Anxious Brain*, and coauthor of *The Panic Workbook for Teens* and *Break Free from Intrusive Thoughts*

"This is an incredibly timely resource from such a talented clinician in our field. What a gift this is to the professional community, as well as to those who suffer with health anxiety. Karen shares her expertise in a validating and relatable way, and those who need help can now get it from one of the best. Thank you, Karen Cassiday!"

—**Beth Salcedo, MD**, psychiatrist and medical director of The Ross Center for Anxiety and Related Disorders, with offices in DC, Northern VA and New York City, NY; and board member of the ADAA

"This book is an amazing gift in times such as these. I know too well how debilitating health anxiety can be, and this is exactly what I needed thirty years ago. Cassiday clearly and compassionately presents valuable context, personal accounts, and science-based therapies to help those struggling build resilience and cultivate peace. This book is the key that will unlock a happier and healthier mindset for countless readers."

—**Wendy Tamis Robbins**, speaker, anxiety coach, attorney, and best-selling author of *The Box*

"An essential resource for anyone overwhelmed by illness concerns, *Freedom from Health Anxiety* is loaded with evidence-based suggestions to help you step away from avoidance, reassurance seeking, and other tactics that counterintuitively make anxiety more difficult to manage. The powerful concepts in this book will help you understand and work through persistent patterns of worry, tolerate the difficult emotions driven by uncertainty, and selectively respond to health concerns in new, more productive ways."

—**Joel Minden, PhD**, licensed clinical psychologist, and author of *Show Your Anxiety Who's Boss*

FREEDOM *from* HEALTH ANXIETY

Understand *and* Overcome Obsessive Worry about Your Health *or* Someone Else's *and* Find Peace *of* Mind

KAREN LYNN CASSIDAY, PhD

New Harbinger Publications, Inc.

Distributed in Canada by Raincoast Books

New Harbinger Publications, Inc.
5674 Shattuck Avenue
Oakland, CA 94609
www.newharbinger.com

Cover design by Amy Daniel

Acquired by Ryan Buresh

Edited by Teja Watson

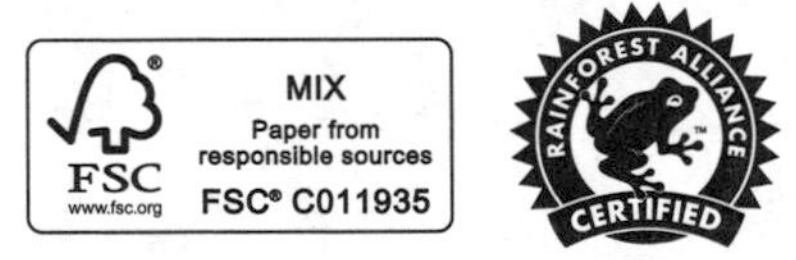

Library of Congress Cataloging-in-Publication Data

Names: Cassiday, Karen, author.
Title: Freedom from health anxiety : understand and overcome obsessive worry about your health or someone else's and find peace of mind / Karen Cassiday, PhD.
Description: Oakland, CA : New Harbinger Publications, Inc., [2022] | Includes bibliographical references.
Identifiers: LCCN 2021047413 | ISBN 9781684039043 (trade paperback)
Subjects: LCSH: Anxiety. | Worry--Prevention. | Stress (Psychology) | Peace of mind. | Mental health. | COVID-19 (Disease)
Classification: LCC BF575.A6 C375 2022 | DDC 152.4/6--dc23
LC record available at https://lccn.loc.gov/2021047413

Printed in the United States of America

24 23 22

10 9 8 7 6 5 4 3 2 1 First Printing

This book is dedicated to everyone who longs for peace of mind as they journey through a life that includes both the potential for great beauty and meaning alongside the certainty of bodily suffering and death.

Contents

Foreword

As I write this in July 2021, the world is approximately eighteen months into the COVID-19 pandemic, which has to date affected 220 countries and territories, with more than 191 million cases and 4 million deaths reported worldwide. In addition to its staggering impact on physical well-being and mortality, large-scale disasters like these are almost always accompanied by increases in mental health disorders, with the mental health footprint typically eventually exceeding the medical one.

Prior to this pandemic, studies on the epidemiology of health anxiety suggested that it is a relatively common condition that, unlike other anxiety disorders that are more prevalent in women, appears to affect men and women equally. There were also already suggestions that rates of health anxiety were increasing, in part due to a more intense focus on monitoring health via smartphones and other connected health devices (activity trackers, Bluetooth-enabled scales and chest-strap heart rate monitors, sleep tracking devices, etc.) and in part due to an increasing use of the Internet to search for medical information for self-diagnosis of concerning symptoms.

With this backdrop in mind, it is easy to imagine health anxiety taking center stage amongst the many medical and mental health consequences of COVID-19. People with health anxiety prior to the pandemic may have experienced an exacerbation in their symptoms, and people without health anxiety prior to the pandemic may now have been primed to interpret bodily sensations and symptoms, no matter how small, as dangerous or potentially even lethal. While both scenarios may be justified and even considered reasonable during this time, we know that once established, health anxiety leads to continued vigilance and is often associated with constant scanning of the body, repeated requests for reassurance, and increased browsing on the Internet, all of which may fuel the vicious cycle by increasing anxiety and intensifying symptoms, leading to catastrophic misinterpretations—even after the pandemic recedes.

Fortunately, highly effective psychological treatments exist for treating health anxiety, with cognitive behavioral therapy (CBT) being the most well-established of the lot, enabling patients to achieve relief from their symptoms that is both rapid and durable. One of the most commonly cited limitations of CBT, however, is the difficulty involved in finding access to an expert mental health provider who is capable of delivering treatment as designed and tested in empirical studies. That is where a book like *Freedom from Health Anxiety* comes in.

Written by Dr. Karen Lynn Cassiday, former president of the Anxiety and Depression Association of America and one of the world's authorities on both CBT and anxiety disorders, *Freedom from Health Anxiety* provides readers with all the skills they need to overcome their health anxiety—be it recent or long-standing, related to the COVID-19 pandemic or some other internal or external trigger. Dr. Cassiday's approach consolidates the latest evidence-based strategies from CBT, along with mindfulness, acceptance, positive psychology, and gratitude, into a step-by-step approach targeting the core problematic areas that experts believe fuel the cycle (negative reinforcement, intolerance of uncertainty, and unhelpful worry-promoting beliefs). Along the way, the book provides a plethora of "raise your resilience" prompts for deeper growth, and is chock-full of success stories that bring to life the concepts covered and help to normalize the prevalence of health anxiety and the powerful impact it can have on our lives.

While I particularly enjoyed her advice on the risks of playing doctor, breaking up with WebMD, and dealing with jargon, Dr. Cassiday also highlights other ways to give up reassurance-seeking and manage a health care system that inadvertently promotes our health anxiety, as well as ways to build tolerance for uncertainty, deal with real health risks, and enhance recovery using exposure to bodily sensations. All of this is presented in a collaborative and validating tone, and even includes personal examples from Dr. Cassiday's life.

As Dr. Cassiday notes, "I know that you don't want to accidentally keep something in your life that has the power to ruin every important aspect of it."

I assume it's no accident that you've picked up this book. Consider yourself fortunate. You now have a chance, with Dr. Cassiday's expert wisdom and guidance, to break the cycle of health anxiety by deliberately choosing to think and act differently, and in so doing, get back to living the life you've always wanted: one that gives you *Freedom from Health Anxiety*. I wish you all the best in your journey and leave you now in the most capable hands of Dr. Karen Cassiday.

—Simon A. Rego, PsyD, ABPP, A-CBT
Chief of Psychology, Montefiore Medical Center
Associate Professor of Psychiatry and Behavioral Sciences, Albert Einstein College of Medicine

CHAPTER 1

When Is Illness Anxiety a Problem?

Do your worries about you or someone you love getting cancer or another serious illness interrupt your life or make you lose sleep? Do you ever wish that other people or the media would stop talking about the tragic illnesses that can kill people because it makes you so anxious? You are not alone. Up to 979 million people in the world experience anxiety about illness that disrupts their lives (Scarella et al. 2019).

Illness anxiety can plague you with painful and convincing worries that you, or someone you love, has a terrible disease and that the end is coming soon. You can spend hours researching symptoms on the Internet, calling doctors, consulting with friends, scanning your body, scanning someone else's body.

Then a doctor discovers that all is well—and you notice a new symptom and do it all over again.

It's exhausting and demoralizing. It makes life feel like walking a tightrope of good health, at risk of falling off at any moment.

You might also have accidentally annoyed your doctor or the people you love with questions about your health or their health. You may even have been reprimanded by your doctor or nurse for repeatedly checking in with them. Maybe they told you that your health is fine, but that you have a problem with anxiety. But you likely pushed this aside, because the thing you saw or felt in your body was real and needs an explanation.

If you are like many people I treat, you are always balancing your desire for good health with your desire to avoid anxiety. But somehow the anxiety always wins out and you end up feeling miserable, only to be repeatedly told by doctors, friends, and family to stop worrying. You might even believe that it is necessary to worry about your health, because you don't want to risk being sloppy with health care, or lack a proper understanding of how to maintain good health. You may consider those who don't worry about their health both admirable because they have peace of mind and foolish because they don't take enough precautions.

Have you considered that perhaps anxiety is the problem? That you might learn to live in peace, knowing that illness can happen to anyone? Even if you are ambivalent about reading this book, I hope you will keep reading—because you deserve the opportunity to enjoy good health without worry. I want to help you feel secure in your good health, by sharing both what it means to have illness anxiety—and how to overcome it, by using scientific strategies that have proven to help.

People with illness anxiety are likely to experience the following range of symptoms (American Psychiatric Association 2013):

- Repeated worry about developing a serious or life-threatening illness
- Repeated attempts to gain reassurance about serious illness by seeking information about illness from health care providers or media
- Feeling anxious and even panicky when thinking about or talking about feared illnesses, despite reassurance from others
- Repeated checking for the presence of symptoms of serious or life-threatening illness
- Feeling preoccupied and unable to concentrate when anxious about a serious or life-threatening illness

What's the Problem with Having Illness Anxiety?

Illness anxiety can make you believe that your worry and repeated checking of symptoms helps you avoid getting serious illness, before it is too late to do something to prevent disability and death. You may think of your anxiety as a protector that keeps you sharp about staying healthy.

But unfortunately, your worry and protective steps don't confer any protection against disease or terminal illness. What they actually do is cripple you with such anxiety that you cannot enjoy your good health. This is backed up by research that shows that when you are uncomfortably anxious about illness, you fail to gain an advantage over people who never worry about their health. In fact, the opposite is true: people who worry about their health engage in fewer health-promoting and serious illness-preventing behaviors than people who don't worry about their health (Ferrer et al. 2013, Amuta et al. 2018).

If you fail to treat your illness anxiety, you run the risk of living with repeated bouts of worry and anxiety, which can disturb both your waking hours and your sleep (Fergus 2016). Many of the people I see report having nightmares about serious illness and terminal illness. You could alienate yourself from those you love and even from your health care providers. Illness anxiety might also drive you to get tests that expose you to unnecessary procedures, exploratory surgeries, treatments, medications, and exposure to radiation (X-rays and CT scans). Your anxious reassurance-seeking could even frustrate your health care providers to the point that they assume all of your symptoms are caused by anxiety, and therefore stop taking your health complaints seriously. This is what happened to Lela. Lela's name is fictitious, and the details of her story have been modified to preserve her privacy. The same is true for all future illustrations of how illness anxiety affects people's lives. Additionally, each person highlighted in this book is someone who overcame their illness anxiety by practicing the strategies described in this book.

Lela's Story

Lela had a close friend die of breast cancer at a young age. This triggered severe worry on Lela's part that she, too, would get breast cancer, because she had many similarities to this close friend.

Lela started by getting a mammogram, which showed all was well. She then worried that cancer could be growing that was undetectable on the first mammogram, so she went to another doctor and got a second mammogram. She did this several more times within the same month, until one of the radiologists happened to talk to another one and realized they had seen the same patient within several days. This radiologist called her and told her to stop getting more mammograms—since getting excessive mammograms was itself creating an elevated risk for getting cancer.

Next, Lela began doing multiple breast self-exams, but she worried that her anxiety made her incapable of identifying any changes. She then turned to her spouse to ask him to check her breasts.

Lela also began worrying that her small child had colon cancer, after he had red flecks in his stool. She called the hospital crisis line and persuaded the pediatrician on call to let her bring in a sample of her son's stool to get checked, even though they did not think it necessary. The results showed that all was well with her son.

She then began calling her son's pediatrician every week, in alarm about her son's stool, which she refused to let her son flush down the toilet, wanting to check it for red flecks. If she thought she saw red, she then took in a stool sample.

The pediatrician banned her from bringing in any more stool samples and told her that she had a problem with anxiety. Her husband reported that he hated having his wife beg him to do her breast exams to check for signs of cancer, and agreed that she had a problem with anxiety. The pediatrician, who knew that I specialize in working with children, teens, and adults who suffer from anxiety and anxiety-related disorders, referred her to me. He also knew that the best treatment for anxiety is exposure-based therapy, which is my specialty—severe and complicated cases that stymie other medical and mental health professionals. He knew that I enjoy working with people like Lela and would not consider her to be a medical nuisance but rather someone who was caught in a trap of anxious reassurance-seeking.

Lela's story illustrates how health worry can grow out of control and disrupt our peace of mind, relationships, and health care.

Refocusing

I know that you don't want to accidentally keep something in your life that has the power to ruin every important aspect of it. I also know that your anxiety makes it feel difficult to turn your focus from scrutinizing your health to examining how you can overcome your worry.

Let's take the first step in the refocusing process, by assessing the negative impact your illness anxiety is having upon your life. Doing so will make it easier to remember why you want to try new thoughts and behaviors when your anxiety gets triggered in the future. It will set the stage for your long-term success with overcoming your illness anxiety.

EXERCISE Assessing the Negative Impact of Your Illness Anxiety

I would like you to take an honest, soul-searching look at how your illness anxiety has negatively affected your life. You can either use a journal or notebook or download worksheets for each of the exercises in this book (available at http://www.newharbinger.com/49043).

Following is a checklist to help you identify the negative effects of your illness anxiety. You may need to fill this out over several days, in order to gently and thoughtfully take stock of all the ways that you are negatively affected. Again, you can download this checklist at http://www.newharbinger.com/49043.

Category	Problems Caused by My Illness Anxiety
Negative Reaction of Others	☐ *Others tell me I worry too much about my health* ☐ *Others get angry or resentful because of my checking for or asking about symptoms* ☐ *I have gotten into arguments with others about illness worries* ☐ *Others have been irritable with me because of my repeated questions about illness worries* ☐ *Others have threatened to cut off contact because of my illness worries*
Feedback from Others	☐ *Others have told me that I have illness issues* ☐ *Someone has told me that I should get treatment for my illness worries* ☐ *Someone gave me this book because they think I worry too much about illness* ☐ *Others have told me that I am a hypochondriac*
Negative Effect on My Daily Life	☐ *I have had trouble concentrating or doing daily tasks because I am so worried about illness* ☐ *My worries about illness have ruined a vacation or other special occasion* ☐ *I hate having medical appointments because I worry so much ahead of time* ☐ *I have lost sleep or eaten too much/too little because of illness worries* ☐ *My illness worries have made me cry or feel emotional* ☐ *I prefer to change the topic of conversation when it turns to illness or death* ☐ *I avoid medical-themed shows because they trigger my illness worries*

Category	Problems Caused by My Illness Anxiety
Checking Behaviors	☐ *When my illness worries get triggered, I check with someone who has medical knowledge or medical experience* ☐ *When my illness anxiety gets triggered, I go on the Internet to get more information about illness* ☐ *When my illness anxiety gets triggered, I check my body, or someone else's, to make sure everything is okay* ☐ *I try to disguise my checking for symptoms of illness so I do not annoy others* ☐ *I own medical equipment that I use to check symptoms that alarm me, even when my doctor has not told me to do this* ☐ *I use medical equipment more than others in the same situation* ☐ *I cannot stop myself from talking about what worries me once my illness worries have been triggered* ☐ *I repeatedly check my body in the shower or bath, to make sure I am okay* ☐ *I take pictures of my symptoms each time I check them, so I can make sure they are not getting worse*

Category	Problems Caused by My Illness Anxiety
Avoidance Behaviors	☐ *I put off medical appointments for fear of getting bad news* ☐ *I avoid finding out the results of medical tests for fear of getting bad news* ☐ *I avoid mention of illnesses, death, or dying because they make me worry* ☐ *I avoid places that remind me of illness, death, or dying* ☐ *I avoid activities that make me think about health*
Financial Cost	☐ *I have spent money on tests, procedures, or consultations that my doctor did not recommend* ☐ *I have spent money repeating a test because of my worries* ☐ *I have spent money on duplicate medical equipment because of my worries*
Other	☐ *I have been reprimanded or lost a job because of absenteeism due to illness anxiety* ☐ *My children have had academic difficulties due to me keeping them home from school in case they are seriously ill*

How did you feel when you went through the checklist above? My guess is that many of these things happen to you on a regular basis. You are suffering, and your suffering is having a negative effect on the people around you.

It's time to take the necessary steps to recover your peace of mind around health. Let's now focus on setting a new goal: for your life without illness anxiety.

Doing the Things that Guarantee Success

If you want to achieve a new goal, you have to know what it is that you're trying to achieve. If you have no idea what success looks like, then you end up randomly trying to figure out what you're supposed to do as you go along. It's like what happens to me when my children ask me to play video games with them. I enter a virtual environment with no instructions, and everyone else seems to know what to do except me, and I end up frustrated.

When the doctor or nurse tells you to stop worrying, it may sound like a good idea—but an impossible one, because you have no idea what tools to use or how to go about getting unstuck from worry. Just as, if my children would give me some clear instructions on how to play the game—besides just handing me the controller and then expecting me to catch on— I might have a chance at making it to the next level.

To overcome your illness anxiety, you need to know what the best strategies are. The chapters that follow will go into depth on the strategies I recommend, which have been proven to help overcome your illness anxiety. Following are some of them, briefly outlined to give you just a taste.

Learn to tolerate scary thoughts and situations. This is an important skill, because no human being can live a life free of risk, bad news, dying, death, or illness. No matter what, life reminds us that we are all mortal beings who live in bodies that get sick, age and die. Since it's impossible to avoid awareness of these facts, the best policy is for us to learn to live in peace and acceptance of these facts.

Learn to tolerate and accept symptoms. Discomfort and the normal fluctuation of body sensations are part of being human. Since it's normal for our bodies to feel a wide range of emotions and physical sensations every day, it's best to make peace with these changes. Even if you have a chronic or serious medical condition, you have to learn to live with fluctuating symptoms.

Learn to live fully in the present moment, instead of in the imagined awful future. None of us knows what exactly will happen in the future, so it's best to enjoy the only thing we have for sure: the present moment. If you want to have robust mental health, then I suggest learning to focus on and enjoy the pleasures of the present, even when challenged by pain, suffering, or knowledge of death. You'll need to learn to focus on things that bring you purpose, meaning, and joy, even if you're facing serious or terminal illness. This may sound impossible at the moment you read this sentence, but I want you to dare to imagine yourself learning to be that kind of courageous and zesty person.

Learn to face and embrace situations that scare you. These situations offer you the opportunity to rapidly overcome your illness anxiety. Your life matters and is most definitely worth the challenge of completing the exercises in this book. You can settle for living with illness anxiety and a severely compromised life, or you can take up the challenge and embrace it.

Let's take a moment for you to imagine how a person who aims toward these goals reacts when they notice a bodily symptom.

MENTAL EXERCISE: Take 5–10 minutes to do this meditation on acceptance, self-compassion, and positive focus.

- Picture yourself in the future, noticing an alarming physical symptom.
- Take the time to accept that it's present, noticing that you're feeling and thinking anxiously.
- Then identify your real enemy—illness anxiety—and remind yourself that you no longer have to do anything because of either your anxiety or your symptom.
- Observe yourself refocusing on something that you enjoy, something that matters or needs to be done, and see yourself engaging with this task or thought.

- As you allow the anxiety to naturally subside, remind yourself that your anxiety often guides you in the wrong direction.
- Keep refocusing on what really matters in this moment and day. Take the time to feel grateful for what is good about your day, your health, and your life at this moment. When your mind returns to your anxiety, remind yourself that you're only human.

Let's now look into why it's so difficult for someone with an anxiety disorder to give up the behaviors that disrupt their life and relationships.

CHAPTER 2

Why Can't I Stop Worrying About My Health?

You have probably asked yourself, "How come I can't stop worrying about my health?" You know that you would like to feel free from anxiety *and* protect your health, or the health of someone you love. You can probably identify with Jacob, who wanted to make sure that he did an excellent job protecting his health.

Jacob's Story

Jacob was a healthy thirty-five-year-old man who began running and lifting weights in high school, after his father had a cardiac catheterization and had to take heart medication. Jacob had learned about family risk factors for heart attacks and stroke in health class. He assumed that he was at increased risk for heart disease because he was a male, and he'd had an early need for reading glasses, like his father had when he was a child. This made Jacob feel that he would follow his father's pattern of physical health—even though his father, unlike Jacob, had never been a regular exerciser, had not done sports in high school, and had smoked cigarettes during his early twenties. Jacob had never smoked and had always eaten a healthy diet.

Jacob began having nightmares about having a heart attack and would wake up panicked, fearing that he was having a heart attack. He began surfing the Internet for information about heart disease and cardiac health. He started wearing a chest band that monitored his heart rate while running, and would slow down his pace if he felt that his heart rate was getting too fast.

Jacob met with his general physician for his annual physical. During the exam, his doctor asked about his family history for heart disease and casually mentioned, "We should keep an eye on your heart because of your father's health history."

This alarmed Jacob. He thought, "Why did he say that? Does he think something is wrong?" He insisted on getting a referral to see a cardiologist, even though his doctor thought this unnecessary.

The cardiologist said that he didn't see a need for any further testing or another visit, because Jacob was in such good health. Jacob felt so worried that he persuaded the cardiologist to conduct a baseline EKG. The night before the EKG, Jacob was so terrified that he would get bad news that he could not sleep. He even wished that he had never seen the cardiologist, because then he would not have to get the test and risk getting bad news.

After he got the EKG, which showed that his heart was healthy, he worried that something was missed, because the EKG took only a few minutes. He then found a very expensive concierge doctor who agreed to give him a treadmill stress test, to check his heart—which was again found to be healthy. He also convinced the concierge doctor to order a Holter monitor, which Jacob wore for a week, to record and report on his heart's activity around the clock, just to make sure that everything was okay. Once again, the results were good, even though there were a few episodes of rapid heartbeats that might have been caused by anxiety. These results further alarmed Jacob.

Jacob's wife became very upset when he began checking his pulse, comparing each side of his neck with each wrist, and keeping records of his various pulse rates. She was also very angry at the money spent on these doctor visits, since it costs thousands of dollars to pay out of pocket for the concierge doctor visit and various unnecessary tests. She eventually called our clinic, because she said that she could no longer talk to him about his health and would leave him if he spent any more money on medical testing and doctors.

Jacob is like many people with illness anxiety who accidentally minimize the impact of their anxiety, because they fear the repercussions of giving up the behaviors that make them feel safe. He falsely believed that he would become even more unbearably anxious if he were to stop checking his heart rate, reading about heart disease, and talking with health care providers about his potential for heart disease. His out-of-control worry convinced him that he needed reassurance each time his worry got triggered: confirmation of good health from his doctor, then again from the cardiologist, and finally from the concierge doctor.

Jacob's story illustrates one of the most frustrating things about having illness anxiety: the more you try to get rid of the anxiety—by seeking reassurance, by avoiding things that make you anxious, by getting expert opinions—the worse it seems to get. You have probably felt like you're going crazy sometimes, because you know that you have illness anxiety and you're doing everything in your power to get past it and prevent another round of worry about health—yet it keeps getting worse. This is common and very understandable, once you learn how anxiety works in your brain and body. Understanding the connection between worry about health, seeking reassurance that all is well, and avoiding things that make you worry will make it much easier to see what must be done to overcome your illness anxiety.

Your Brain Pays Attention to Scary Things First

First, it's important to understand that your brain and body are hardwired to process information about danger and fear first. Your brain can process fear-related information faster than you can think, in the lower and middle parts that don't rely upon thought or decision-making. This is very helpful when real danger presents itself, such as seeing a car that crosses a lane into your path. Your brain allows you to react rapidly, without having to think about the situation. When your life is threatened by real danger, you need to be able to do something fast, such as swerving to avoid the oncoming traffic.

The problem with your brain is that it cannot distinguish between real danger and imagined danger. It's hardwired to assume that anything that resembles danger, whether real or imagined, is important—and therefore triggers an alarm signal. The alarm signal is the same for every situation. It's the reason that your heart beats fast, and you breathe more quickly and feel shaky when you watch a scary scene in a movie or ride a roller coaster, both of which are safe activities. Your brain and nervous system react as though the danger is terrible and real, and they activate your mind and body. The symptoms in your body prepare you for the imagined emergency. This response is also a sort of "on/off" switch, with no way to give a graduated response. Your body gives the same level of activation if you see a pretend grizzly bear in a movie as it does if you see a large, angry grizzly bear while camping in the mountains. It just happens.

We also know that if many of your relatives and ancestors tended to worry and get anxious, you probably tend to worry and get anxious too. Evidence shows that one of the things that runs in families who experience anxiety disorders is the genetic tendency to overreact to stressors and to things that provoke anxiety (McGregor et al. 2018). The process by which chemicals associated with fear and anxiety get activated and then return to a resting state in families can be more easily disrupted in some, and less easily in others. We also know that families whose members suffer from anxiety are more likely to accidentally promote the behaviors that make anxiety worse, such as avoiding things that trigger anxiety. This makes it difficult for children to learn how to face and manage anxious feelings.

Elders in the families of those who experience anxiety may also show children that uncertainty about life is something to worry about, and may act as though you can only trust expert opinions, and never your own. That sets you up for feeling unnecessary doubt. Also, these families might accidentally promote the idea that anxiety is something terrible and is best avoided, rather than teaching children that anxiety is a common and manageable emotion. If you came from one of these kinds of families, then you likely witnessed other people who were more anxious and worried than other people's relatives. You may have not been taught the set of skills you need to handle your tendency to get anxious about illness. Here is what Jenna said about how her upbringing made her sensitive to illness anxiety.

Jenna's Story

My earliest memories of my grandparents were of my family constantly worrying that they would die. My grandmother was always calling for an ambulance because she feared that she or my grandfather were dying. She would always say goodbye to us grandkids saying, "If the blessed Virgin lets me live that long." She and my dad went to the doctor for everything, whether it was a cold, sore foot, or scratchy throat.

I can barely recall a night that I did not get my forehead checked to make sure I was not sick. All the grown-ups would tell me, "Don't get sweated up. You might get sick." Getting sick was something awful that required lots of doctor visits, prayers, and lit candles for God's mercy. I stayed home from school even when I did not want to because my mom worried that I might be sick and make things worse.

If someone actually was sick, then everyone talked to everyone else in the whole family about it and worried together about whether or not the person who had a cold or a cough would get seriously ill. I can hardly remember anyone praying for things other than sparing people from illness and death. I was so surprised when I learned in junior high school that other people sent their kids to school or let them play outdoors while they had a runny nose or cough.

You can see from Jenna's story how easy it might be to learn unhelpful ways to think and act when it comes to feeling unwell or being sick. She had lots of opportunities to accidentally make anxiety worse and very few to see how to avoid the trap of worry and reassurance-seeking that plagued her family.

The Role of Negative Reinforcement in Your Illness Anxiety

These conditions can make it very easy for you to get caught up in a cycle of negative reinforcement. Negative reinforcement is what happens when you get anxious and you try to quickly get rid of your anxiety, instead of letting it naturally subside. It's the anxiety equivalent of giving in to a toddler who has a tantrum, because you cannot stand to hear the toddler cry. The more you give in to the toddler's tantrum, the more the toddler cries and demands your attention.

Just like a toddler who tantrums, your anxiety grabs your attention and fools you into thinking that it's an emergency, and that you cannot manage the moment unless you give in to the urge to get immediate relief. You might try to get reassurance by talking to a friend, to see if they have had similar symptoms; or by talking to a doctor or nurse to get their opinion; or looking up information about illness, to make sure you don't have symptoms that coincide with a serious illness; or trying to get a medical test, to prove nothing is wrong.

Then, each time that you give in to this urge, you guarantee that you will feel more anxiety the *next* time you encounter something that makes you think about illness—whether it's noticing a symptom, checking your body, checking someone else's body, or overhearing something that makes you think about illness. Thus, the more you check, read about illness, visit your doctor, or avoid things that make you think about illness, the more you feed your anxiety disorder. This is the process of negative reinforcement.

Another thing negative reinforcement does is make it seem necessary to check your body for signs of dangerous illness—or to check someone else's body. Scanning for symptoms rapidly reduces the anxiety about wondering whether or not there's something alarming happening with your health. Every time you check, you make it more likely that you will feel driven to check again, the next time you get a scary thought about illness. You also accidentally reinforce your mind, developing a high-alert system for noticing any potential signs of illness.

Therapists call this becoming hypervigilant. The more hypervigilant you become, the more things you notice—whether it's bumps on your skin, lumps in your body, odd moles on your skin, strange sensations, changes in your vision, weird aches, changes in your stool, or unexplained headaches. The more you think about frightening symptoms and notice potential signs of illness in your body, the more your anxiety increases, because of the process of negative reinforcement.

Then, unfortunately, the experience of anxiety creates a host of symptoms that are often misinterpreted as further proof of possible illness: fatigue, poor sleep, feeling achy, headaches, stomachaches, upset stomach, feeling restless, feeling dizzy, poor concentration, increased heart rate, sweating, trembling, and feeling faint. All of which can be found on any list of symptoms of rare and serious illnesses on the Internet (Wilson 2009).

There's another problem. Repeated examination of symptoms can also create pain, swelling, and bruising. If you keep touching, poking, or prodding areas of your body that are concerning to you, you can make them look and feel worse —and even more alarming. You might even take photos of various parts of your body, your stool, your sputum, or other things, to try and determine whether or not alarming changes have occurred. Then, it gets more difficult to determine if there is a significant difference, which in turn elevates your anxiety, which makes it seem even more important to take more photos and scrutinize them. In summary, all the things you think and do to immediately make yourself feel better backfire and make your anxiety much worse. Gerry's story illustrates how hypervigilance and checking can make illness anxiety worse.

Gerry's Story

Gerry had a close friend die of testicular cancer shortly after college. While his friend was dying, he made Gerry promise to do consistent self-checking of his testicles so that he would not suffer the same fate.

Gerry also read up on his friend's symptoms and learned that many men miss the early symptoms, when treatment is more likely to succeed, and may only notice their cancer once it spreads. He then began a monthly routine of checking his entire body for any unusual lumps, bumps, or indentations, especially in his genitals and the lymph nodes in his groin, armpits, and neck.

Monthly checking soon became weekly checking, which turned into daily checking, with multiple selfies of areas of concern. The more Gerry checked, the more confused he became about what he had detected in previous checks, since there were so many episodes of checking. The areas he checked also sometimes became sore or swollen, because he would press firmly and pinch the skin to try and determine if what he felt was a true hard mass that might indicate cancer, or just a swollen area due to a benign illness.

Gerry also studied self-check videos, to make sure his technique was correct, and then rechecked to make sure he had done it right. When his armpits, neck, and groin felt sore, he became even more anxious and in need of repeat checking, in case this meant the cancer was rapidly growing. He even had occasional bruising, due to overly vigorous self-checks.

The more uncertain he felt about what he noticed, the more he checked, and the more he doubted his technique and what he detected. The more anxious and worried he felt, the less he slept and felt like eating. The less he ate, the more nauseous he felt. Feeling nauseous and fatigued then exacerbated his fear that he really must have cancer, because he was young, fit, and supposed to be feeling healthy instead of sickly.

He felt terrified that he might be dying but also knew that he did not have symptoms that necessitated a doctor appointment. He finally started treatment with me after a work supervisor asked him if something was wrong because he spent so much time in the restroom checking while at work.

EXERCISE Identifying the Negative Reinforcers of Your Illness Anxiety

Get out your journal or notebook. Think about your personal negative reinforcers. These are all the mental and behavioral activities that you do to try and quickly reduce anxiety about illness, without simply allowing your anxiety to return to baseline of its own accord.

Save this list, because you will use it when we work on overcoming your illness anxiety disorder. Below is a sample list of different ways that people with illness anxiety disorder engage in negative reinforcement, to get you started. A worksheet for this exercise is available at http://www.newharbinger.com/49043.

- *Researching symptoms when I notice a symptom or worry about a symptom*
- *Asking others for their opinion about a symptom or a disorder*
- *Repeatedly asking similar questions to my doctor/nurse about a symptom or disorder after they tell me not to worry*
- *Repeatedly emailing, texting, or calling my doctor/nurse when I am worried about a symptom*
- *Asking my doctor/nurse for tests, procedures, or surgery when they did not first suggest a test or procedure*
- *Calling the after-hours medical hotline to ask about a worrisome symptom because I could not wait until the next open office hours*
- *Checking with multiple doctors/nurses about the same symptoms and getting extra consultations just to make sure everything is okay*
- *Repeatedly discussing what my doctor/nurse said to me with others, to make sure it sounds accurate*
- *Researching the information my doctor/nurse gave me to make sure it's correct*
- *Getting repeated tests for the same symptom even though the first test result was okay*

- *Repeatedly checking my body, or that of someone I love, for signs of serious illness, or serious change in illness status*
- *Repeatedly checking health care information to make sure that I understood it correctly*
- *Checking my body so much that it gets sore, irritated, or swollen*
- *If I have a symptom, repeatedly checking it, e.g., checking temperature every fifteen minutes, checking pulses on both sides of neck, both wrists, and both ankles*
- *Asking my doctor/nurse to check a symptom again after it has already been checked*
- *Repeatedly checking what I ate or did to make sure that it explains changes in how I feel, e.g., that my sweating is due to eating spicy food, instead of a serious illness*

Writing down *your* personal list of negative reinforcers might feel difficult, because you might think of them as your go-to strategies for feeling better. Properly identifying the things that trap you in continued illness anxiety takes courage and humility, to recognize that what you have been doing is counterproductive.

You may find as you read through the following chapters that you discover more negative reinforcers than you first recognized. Please be patient with yourself and your recovery. It takes time to recognize how your anxiety has pushed you into a dead end of worry. The good news is, the better you become at identifying your negative reinforcers, the sooner you can practice the skills that lead to peace of mind and long-term recovery.

The Danger of Avoidance

Avoiding situations that make you worry is another form of negative reinforcement. Each time you try to stop thinking about serious illness, try to stop others from talking about it, avoid media that reminds you of it, avoid getting medical tests, avoid encounters with health care professionals, or avoid hospitals or medical facilities, you reinforce all of the anxiety and worry that led to the aversion. This behavior only guarantees that you'll feel even more frightened the next time you encounter these situations. It also gives credence to the belief that you can't handle what makes you anxious, because you put off opportunities to gain mastery over your fears. Avoidance always backfires when it comes to anxiety, because it never allows you the chance to discover how strong you can be in the face of anxiety.

You may feel like it's cruel or foolish to stop avoiding the things that trigger your illness anxiety. If you do, it's likely because you feel unable to do anything about the onslaught of worry and anxiety that immediately follows getting triggered. Please dare to believe that you can become powerful in your ability to overcome your illness anxiety.

When you learn the science-proven strategies that this book describes, you can begin to think of the situations and thoughts that you avoid as opportunities for growth and mastering your body's anxious response to triggers. You will have to learn to reframe your brain's automatic alarm signal as a signal to use your newly learned skills.

EXERCISE Identifying the Ways Illness Anxiety Makes You Avoidant

Let's spend some time identifying the ways in which your illness anxiety makes you avoid thoughts and activities that you would otherwise tolerate or enjoy. Put your answers in your notebook or journal, for future reference when we work on overcoming your illness anxiety disorder.

You can borrow items from the previous list you made of the negative impact of your illness anxiety. Also, try to list things that people without illness anxiety do easily, even though you may believe that you need to do these things to remain safe and healthy. If you follow the exercises described in this book, you will begin to doubt the wisdom of avoiding these things and become willing to live a life that has more freedom from illness anxiety. Here is a sample list of avoidant thoughts and behaviors:

- *I avoid thinking about or saying words that remind me of feared illnesses.*
- *I cover my ears, leave the room, or interrupt the conversation when others talk about serious illness.*
- *I avoid attending funerals, visiting hospitals or hospices.*
- *I avoid or delay medical appointments.*
- *I avoid hearing about fundraisers for certain illnesses.*
- *I avoid or delay getting medical tests.*
- *I turn off the TV or other media if the news contains something about an illness I fear.*
- *I cannot finish books that have characters in them that might die of a serious illness.*
- *I avoid religious services that mention death or people dying.*
- *I avoid health assessments, e.g., blood pressure, heart rate, temperature, breast self-exam.*
- *I avoid looking at my body in the mirror because I fear I will find a serious symptom.*
- *I avoid activities that might make me worry about illness, such as exercise, sex, or lifting weights.*
- *I avoid eating certain foods, for fear that they will make me die from a serious illness, such as cancer or heart disease.*
- *I avoid others who have serious illnesses.*
- *I avoid eating foods that might give me symptoms that could be confused with illness, such as caffeinated beverages or spicy foods.*
- *I avoid doing things for fear of catching a serious illness.*

You just took another important step forward in your recovery, by identifying the ways that illness anxiety makes you avoid situations that others without illness anxiety can do. Don't be discouraged if you find that you need to add things to this list as you progress through the exercises in this book. Your point of view about what is necessary to avoid will change as you decrease your anxiety and do more exposure practice, as described in Chapter 3.

Intolerance of Uncertainty

A dislike of uncertainty, or of not knowing what is going to happen, is called *intolerance of uncertainty*. There's a very good chance that you have an elevated level of intolerance of uncertainty. Researchers who study worry have discovered that people who dislike uncertainty are more likely to worry (Dugas, Gosselin, and Ladouceur 2001). People who worry about their health prefer to feel absolutely confident that no terrible illnesses will befall themselves or the people they love.

If you have intolerance of uncertainty, then it's likely that you have had thoughts such as, "I would rather just know that I have cancer, instead of having to not know and wait for my exam results to come back." You might also think, "I am okay as long as I know what I am dealing with. I just cannot cope with not knowing."

You might feel like you handle a crisis well, even a medical crisis, but you fall apart when you feel unsure about whether or not a serious illness is creeping up on you or someone you love. I have had patients say seemingly contradictory statements such as, "I could not take it if I had cancer, but I just want the doctor to hurry up and call me back with the bad news because I cannot take another minute of waiting! I just want to get the bad news over with!"

If you have severe intolerance of uncertainty, you're more likely to dread getting annual physicals and medical tests, because you have to wait to get the results, which your worry convinces you might be very bad news. Remember, one reason your imagined awful news feels so real is because your brain is sending out a full alert signal to your body, because it cannot distinguish between what is real and the imagined awful future.

Intolerance of certainty can become a problem because you narrow your focus from the total range of possibilities (getting good results back from a test, getting ambiguous results back from a test, getting bad results back from a test) to only the negative possibilities (getting bad results).

When you narrow your focus to only scary and terrible things, this reflects your brain's hardwired preference for negative and frightening information, and your desire for a "better safe than sorry" approach to thinking about the future. When you think about only the negative possibilities, your brain and body react to this imagined awful future as though it's a real event, unable to distinguish between real and imagined danger.

Once your body feels anxious, your mind takes this information as confirmation of bad news, without even getting the doctor's diagnosis. You then feel that you're justified in your worry about getting bad news. Do you see how easy it is to get caught in a trap of worry, reassurance-seeking, and avoiding?

EXERCISE Identifying Your Intolerance of Uncertainty

People with intolerance of uncertainty and illness anxiety disorder tend to have thoughts like the ones listed below. If you notice that these thoughts sound like you, please write them down in your journal, so you can keep them in mind when you're working on overcoming your illness anxiety. These thoughts are unhelpful, so you'll want to replace them with helpful thoughts that remind you that uncertainty is a normal part of life. We'll learn more about how to replace these thoughts later in this chapter.

- *I would rather get bad news than wait any longer for my test results.*
- *If a test result is delayed or takes longer than I expected, that must mean it's bad news.*
- *I dread having to wait for my lab results, X-ray results, or for my scans to be read.*
- *It's easier to deal with bad news than to not know what is going on with my symptoms, or the symptoms of someone I love.*

- *It's unfair that there are no guarantees of good health or a long life.*
- *I cannot relax when things are uncertain about my health or the health of someone I love.*
- *I don't like surprising symptoms or changes in my body. I wish things would stay the same.*

Your Worry-Promoting Beliefs

Worry-promoting beliefs can accidentally give you permission to do all the aforementioned behaviors, even when a doctor or therapist has instructed you to stop calling, researching, and checking or avoiding. You might be one of these people if you repeatedly make excuses to indulge in negative reinforcers—for example, going on WebMD every time you worry about an illness, even when you know that your checking, reassurance-seeking, and talking to doctors is fruitless and even harmful. Research has shown that the people who check medical information on the Internet the most are the ones with the highest level of intolerance of uncertainty (Fergus 2015).

This can happen because you've convinced yourself that you're stacking the odds in your favor by checking for more information that might lead to news that gives you reassurance. Many of my patients argue the point that they are keeping themselves or their loved ones extra safe, because they pay such close and careful attention to their health. They make exceptions to their doctor's recommendations for routine visits, screenings, and discussion, because their anxiety over-focuses on risk and danger, and ignores all the good information, such as the doctor's reassurance that there's no need for alarm. They end up, in effect, practicing medicine without a license, because they allow their anxiety to supersede their licensed and well-trained doctor or nurse's advice. And practicing medicine without a license is illegal!

Another reason people justify giving in to reassurance-seeking behavior is by thinking, "This time it really is serious! I might have been lucky up until this point, but now my time is up and this time it's real." They fail to realize that the bias in their brain and body, which mistakes each anxiety alarm as being unique and dangerous, is fooling them into believing that each episode of worry is a signal of true danger, or a serious illness. It's very common, early in treatment, for my patients to tell me, "This time it's different. What if it really is cancer this time?"

Don't be fooled by this feeling that your luck is up, and that the current episode of intense worry and anxiety is a premonition of imminent serious illness. This is just a symptom of having illness anxiety and is common to almost everyone who shares your symptoms. If you recall, one of the characteristics of anxiety is to convince you, "This time it is real! This situation is new, dangerous, and unlike any other you have experienced!" Don't be fooled by this sense of anxious urgency, priority, and novelty. Here is a sample list of typical worry-promoting beliefs that people with illness anxiety disorder often assume are true.

EXERCISE Identifying Your Worry-Promoting Beliefs

Please write down your worry-promoting beliefs in your notebook or journal, so you have them on hand to target in treatment. Your long-term goal is to change these unhelpful beliefs into adaptive and helpful ones that allow for the uncertainty of life.

Take note of your worry-promoting beliefs from the list below, so you have them on hand to target in treatment. Add any worry-promoting beliefs that trigger your illness anxiety or worry in general.A worksheet for this exercise is available at http://www.newharbinger.com/49043.

- ☐ People who worry about their health are more likely to prevent a serious illness and are less likely to die from a serious illness.
- ☐ If I have a strong feeling or premonition that something is seriously wrong with me, or with someone I love, then it's likely to be true.
- ☐ Better safe than sorry. It's always a good idea to check something out.

- ☐ You can never afford to take your health, or someone else's, for granted.
- ☐ It's always best to have an expert check your symptoms. You can never be too careful.
- ☐ You never know when disaster will strike so it's best to be ready.
- ☐ People who do not follow up by checking things out are much more likely to get sick or die.
- ☐ Researching various serious illnesses makes it more likely that you'll prevent a tragedy.
- ☐ Someone has to worry about my, or someone else's, health. It might as well be me. It is a parent's/child's/sibling's/spouse's job to worry about their loved one's health.

What Illness Anxiety Is Not

You might have heard a therapist or doctor suggest that the reason you get so worried about getting seriously ill is because some subconscious part of you wants to be taken care of, or believes that the only legitimate way you can ask for help and comfort is by being sick. This is called *secondary gain*, or the unconscious need to use one set of behaviors to get attention or love from other people, when you don't feel able to get your emotional needs met by your partner, family, or friends.

Therapists used to believe that many people with anxiety disorders, and especially people who worried about illness and accidentally overused the medical system, must suffer from secondary gain (Davidhizar 1994). The good news is that research has shown that this is not true, and that other things—such as how your brain prioritizes processing of fear-related information, genetic predisposition for anxiety disorders, the process of negative reinforcement, and intolerance of uncertainty—are the reasons that people get illness anxiety. Once you understand how the brain and body work, it's easy to see how someone like you can develop this problem.

Some people believe that people with illness anxiety have a need to be sick because they don't want to face up to the pressures and responsibilities of their lives. The idea is that if you can find an illness, then you can get a free pass from having to work, go to school, or deal with annoying people. This too has been shown not to hold up to the test of science.

People with illness anxiety are terrified of being ill and desperately want to be able to live their lives without anxiety. They fear all the illnesses that would take away from their ability to live fully or to be alive. Secondary gain is the last thing on their minds; they would much rather be healthy. This explanation also fails to take into account how the brain and body work when a false alarm of danger is triggered.

You might also have heard people talk about Munchausen Syndrome. This disorder occurs when someone who is healthy deliberately induces an illness or a need for surgery, in order to get medical attention. They might ingest poison, swallow metal implements, or take inappropriate medications that make them very ill, in order to be hospitalized. In this case, the patient does not fear illness, but in fact welcomes the idea of becoming ill, so they can receive the care and attention of medical staff.

People with illness anxiety seek the advice of medical staff to allay their fears, but never with the hope that they will actually come to need treatment for a serious illness. They are, in fact, hoping very much to hear that their health is excellent and that they are in no danger of serious illness.

Now that you understand what causes and maintains illness anxiety, you're ready to learn about how to recover from it. You have identified all the ways that your anxiety interferes with your life, and all the beliefs that make it harder to get rid of your anxiety. In the next chapter we will talk about how to dismantle anxiety-promoting behaviors, by teaching your body and mind how to tolerate anxiety, without giving in to the behaviors that make it worse.

CHAPTER 3

Dealing with Your Fears of Illness, Dying, and Death

Have you ever wondered how you could possibly handle it if you really did get the terrible news that you had a terminal illness? Some years ago, I had the privilege of working on an oncology unit with people who had cancer. Most of them had cancers that at that time were untreatable, and so their care was geared toward lengthening the time that they had left.

Much to my surprise, I learned that many of my patients with untreatable or terminal illnesses were determined to live well and enjoy their lives, even though they knew for sure that death was imminent. When I led the oncology support group, the biggest complaint I heard from terminally ill patients was that they hated it when others would not openly acknowledge that they were dying. They were frustrated that their family members and friends were surprised that they wanted to do as many fun and meaningful things as possible, instead of worrying about dying. One man told me, "I am going to live as much as I can, every day that I can, because I am not dead yet!"

The group members also told me at the start of one group that on that particular day they didn't want to talk about anything to do with cancer, the hospital, or dying—all they wanted to do was to eat some excellent watermelon that a patient's brother had snuck into the ward. So that is exactly what we did! This was fun, full of laughter and good humor.

The group were also full of zest for living, playing jokes on each other and the staff and doing everything they could to enjoy their day. They took every possible opportunity to do ordinary things that they no longer took for granted, such as eating perfectly ripe watermelon, fresh and sweet off the vine.

The reality for many terminally ill people is that their life creates automatic exposure therapy to the awareness of mortality and the inevitability of dying. Many of these patients adapt to this awareness and get practical about living the best lives they can, because they know their time is limited.

This is in direct contradiction to what your anxiety suggests will happen. Your anxiety fails to assure you that you have a remarkable capacity for adapting, learning, and growing, even under the most difficult of circumstances. Anxiety overlooks your ability to become resilient, through practice handling difficult situations. Anxiety, in short, lies to you about your human nature and your ability to become its master.

If you want to overcome your anxiety about illness, dying, and death, then you're going to have to learn how to dismantle the system of negative reinforcement, intolerance of uncertainty, and unhelpful beliefs that set you up for having difficulty in the first place. If you're like most people with this disorder, you're hoping that I will have a method for recovery that leads straight into relaxation, peace of mind, and calm confidence, with no scary thoughts about illness, no scary symptoms, and no terrible diseases or early deaths.

That sounds like a logical goal, but it's off-track, because it doesn't allow for the inevitable reality of life in a human body.

A better goal for treatment is to take into account that random physical symptoms, and sometimes even serious illness or death, are an inevitable part of life. It's better to learn to accept this reality of being human, and to react with a calm, resilient, wise mind when faced with the reality of living in a mortal human body. You're going to have to learn some key life skills that will help you master your anxiety and learn to live with peace of mind.

The best method for overcoming your disorder involves several key components that research has shown work very well, whether you're new to illness anxiety or cannot recall a time in your life when you didn't have it.

Exposure therapy, and a newer enhancement of exposure therapy called *learned inhibition*, is the first key component to becoming a master of self-directed healing from illness anxiety. The following chapters will address other key components that are necessary for your robust recovery.

Exposure Therapy

Exposure therapy has been applied toward the successful treatment of anxiety disorders since the 1980s (Parker et al. 2018). It involves facing your feared thoughts and situations and maintaining these thoughts or staying in these situations repeatedly, until your anxiety naturally subsides on its own. It's the therapy equivalent of riding a scary roller-coaster a hundred times in a row. During the first five to ten rides, you feel terrified, but then you start to feel less afraid, until you get used to it and even feel bored during the last thirty rides.

This process of getting used to something that scares you is called *habituation*. All people and animals have a built-in ability to habituate to things they fear, if they keep repeating the exposure to the thing that is frightening. This happens because the receptors for the fear chemicals in your brain and body get saturated after a few minutes during exposure, and have to shut down until they can receive another dose of fear chemical. Even though your mind might fear an ever-escalating cycle of anxiety, your brain and body have a limit. So, even though you may fear that your anxiety will get much worse if you were to stop checking, stop getting reassurance, or stop talking to your doctor, your anxiety has a ceiling, or limit, and you cannot make it worse.

The feeling of going insane or of losing of control is a symptom of your elevated anxiety. This means that the biggest dilemma for your mind, when your body gets anxious, is its misperception that your anxiety will continue to escalate and that you will not be able to handle your anxiety.

Exposure therapy takes advantage of this natural process of habituation and uses it to your advantage. Typical exposure therapy involves creating a ladder of situations and thoughts to practice, from easiest to most difficult, and then systematically practicing these "exposures" until your anxiety subsides by at least half.

Recent research has shown, however, that there are limitations to conducting exposure therapy this way (Jacoby 2016, Tolin 2019). Sometimes sticking to a ladder of exposure practice that goes from easiest to most difficult makes it easy to assume that doing the most difficult exposure practice is something special and not for every day. People can get content with doing easier practice and delaying the difficult practice until they feel very motivated and prepared.

This is a problem, because life does not present things that create anxiety in a hierarchical fashion that waits until you feel really prepared for difficulties. Often it is quite the opposite! Practicing exposures in a random fashion better mimics what happens in a person's life. It better prepares you to be ready for anything, by learning that you can handle even the most anxiety-provoking situations, whether or not you feel ready. It guarantees that you learn that you can master anxiety, regardless of its seeming power to frighten you.

This chapter will teach you how science shows that you can achieve this.

Creating New Neural Pathways

Research on what happens to the brain during any kind of learning, such as recovering from an anxiety disorder, gives us clues about what might be a new way to enhance treatment for people like you. Brain scans show that when people with anxiety disorders recover, they build new neural pathways for non-anxious thoughts and behaviors. But all the old pathways associated with negative reinforcement and avoidance still remain. That means that any time you learn to do something new, you still remember how to do the unhelpful thoughts and behaviors that maintain your anxiety.

This also explains why it's so easy to relapse and why it can take so long to make new behaviors and thoughts automatic when you're recovering from anxiety about illness. It's the psychological equivalent of remembering to take a new route to work after you have used an old route for years. If you don't pay attention, you accidentally take the turnoff for the old route, until the new route becomes a habit.

If you recall from the previous chapter, your brain prioritizes negative and fear-related information and prefers easy overlearned behaviors to new effortful ones when under duress, e.g., anxiety. This explains why it's easier for you to slip into old unhelpful thoughts and behaviors when you feel anxious, even when you planned to try something else. You're under stress and have not yet practiced enough to make it possible to do the new, more difficult thing.

Anxiety disorder experts therefore realized that a new approach needed to be taken, one that took into account how the brain prioritizes negative and fear-related information. This approach is called *inhibitory learning* (Jacoby 2016, Craske et al. 2014).

If you really want to ramp up the quality of your recovery, you'll want to learn how to suppress, or inhibit, the old thoughts and behaviors that set you up for negative reinforcement, such as seeking reassurance and avoiding. You'll want to work hard to prove to yourself that you can stand firm in the face of fear, no matter what level or symptoms of anxiety you experience. It also means that you'll be simulating, with your recovery program, what happens in real life. Instead of focusing on following an easy-to-difficult ladder of exposures, you'll be focusing on how to accept, embrace, and bring on anxiety-provoking moments, while learning to manage the surprise of random exposure to anxiety-provoking things. You'll pay close attention to cultivating your sense of mastery over the experience of anxiety, and to learning to tolerate risk and uncertainty. You'll simulate the randomness of how anxiety enters your life and coach yourself to be able to handle all of your anxiety symptoms every time, whether you feel weak or strong. Finally, you'll focus on becoming aware of the beliefs and thoughts that impede your ability to face your fear—and you will systematically challenge these beliefs and thoughts. You'll become confident *in your ability to handle your anxiety,* as opposed to being confident that you'll never get anxious again.

No one has discovered a technique to prevent anxiety from occurring. Therefore, your best strategy is to become calm and confident about being able to handle the inevitable moments of anxiety. The paradox is that once you learn to be confident about handling your anxiety and stop engaging in negative reinforcement, your overall level of anxiety will indeed decrease. Your tendency to get worried about your health, however, may always be likely to pop up when you're especially stressed, tired, or ill.

If you suffer from a serious or terminal illness, upsetting moments will no doubt be ahead—and you'll want to have the ability to face these challenges without extreme anxiety and worry. If you focus on the skills in this book, you can prepare yourself to live well for the rest of your life, no matter what.

How to Guarantee Your Exposure Practice Works

There are some rules to follow if you want to make your exposure practice lead to full recovery. Research on exposure-based therapies and inhibitory learning show that you need to address the following things to make your practice powerful.

1. Exposure practice has to make you *feel* your worry and anxiety about illness. If it doesn't make you anxious, then it's not exposure practice. It's necessary to make your body and brain feel the fear that your illness anxiety causes, in order to learn a new way to handle these sensations and thoughts. It's also necessary to feel your anxiety, so you can get used to it and learn to trust that you can handle these sensations and thoughts, even when they are strong. You'll also learn that even when you do nothing, your discomfort will decrease, because your body and brain cannot maintain a constant level of fear or escalate the level of fear once your body's receptors for fear chemicals are saturated. You'll be *learning to tolerate anxiety,* as opposed to getting rid of all anxiety.

2. Exposure practice has to have surprises, because life is unpredictable. You need to teach your body and mind that they can handle the random rough and tumble of unexpected thoughts and sensations that comprise your illness anxiety. Anxiety falsely makes you think that you cannot handle the unexpected. Good treatment teaches you "Yes, you can!"

3. You have to practice embracing risk and uncertainty, because this is a normal part of life and a normal part of your worry about illness. This means that you'll be practicing getting used to the possibility of getting seriously ill, or accepting the serious illness of someone you love. You'll get used to the idea of dying and death and/or accepting the serious or chronic illness that you might already have. You'll have to practice this until you have the same tolerance that non-anxious people do about the possibility of serious illness, dying, and death.

4. You'll have to practice exposure to all of the sensations, thoughts, and situations that accompany your illness anxiety disorder, and to combine these sensations, thoughts, and situations together to make your exposure work well. You must be willing to be thorough, so you can nip all the likely triggers for your illness anxiety. Your goal is to become inoculated against the power of your triggers to provoke your illness anxiety.

5. You'll need to identify the ways in which your illness anxiety disorder creates unhelpful expectations and beliefs about your ability to manage your anxiety, and then use your exposure practice to prove to yourself that these unhelpful expectations and beliefs are sabotaging and no longer apply to you.

6. You'll have to switch into a courageous, risk-taking, adventure-seeking mindset, once you decide that your old safety-oriented, comfort-seeking mindset prevents you from living a full, authentic life without regrets.

7. You'll need to practice as frequently as possible, preferably every day. Once you begin to practice a certain item on your list, you need to make turning back to the old way of avoiding, seeking reassurance, or using that particular method of quick escape for your anxiety a nonnegotiable deletion from your repertoire of choices.

8. You should keep doing your exposure practice until it becomes easy to do and no longer creates anxiety. For some of the practices, this will mean not giving in to an urge to check or seek reassurance. For other practices, it will mean doing something, such as scheduling a doctor's appointment or sticking with a plan. Other exposures may require chunks of time, for repeating feared words or imagining scary scenarios, every day for many days or weeks until these no longer make you anxious. This means that on some days, your exposure practice might take relatively little time, and on other days you may need an hour or two to successfully complete your exposures.

Note: If you're doing exposure to movies or TV shows that trigger your illness anxiety, you can save some time by just watching the scenes that frighten you the most, instead of having to watch the entire movie or show over and over. Additionally, many movies have clips of famous scenes, such as dying or death scenes, on YouTube, so you can try searching for relevant scenes instead of having to watch or rent the entire movie or show.

Your Exposure Practice: Challenging Your Mindset and Unhelpful Beliefs

Please don't make the mistake of taking a passive approach to your exposure therapy. If you approach the task of facing feared situations and thoughts as something to be endured, because you hope it will automatically lead to a reduction in anxiety and get rid of your worry, then you're misguided. Taking a "just get through it" approach dampens the effect of your exposure therapy, because you cling to the hope of living a life that excludes the experience of anxiety. If you do, you may find yourself being able to do all of the behaviors that are on your list, but feeling disappointed because you're still anxious or scared of novel triggers. This is because you took a fearful approach to doing your exposure practice, instead of diving in.

You must perceive the magnificence of discovering that you can handle your worst anxiety, and therefore no longer need fear the experience of anxiety. Wouldn't that be wonderful, to no longer fear getting anxious? Full recovery doesn't mean the absence of anxiety. It means no longer fearing the experience of anxiety, because you know that it's a false signal. It means embracing the human experience of getting anxious as being one of the many experiences that are part of a full, rich life.

With a few rare exceptions, all humans will feel anxiety at different points throughout their life. The people who accept and learn to calmly handle the experience of anxiety are the people who have the mental health advantage. Exposure therapy is one of the best ways to develop and discover your ability to handle and accept the human experience of anxiety.

Anxiety Sensitivity

One of the differences between people with anxiety disorders and those without is that people with anxiety disorders often have an elevated level of *anxiety sensitivity*, or fear of being afraid (Riess et al. 1986). If you have elevated anxiety sensitivity, you may accidentally believe that it's psychologically harmful to feel anxious. You may live to avoid feeling anxious. You may accidentally react to feeling anxious as though it's a catastrophe, instead of considering it to be a mere signal that something has tripped your alarm system.

If you're low in anxiety sensitivity, then you don't dread feeling anxious; maybe you think of feeling anxious as a signal that something is challenging or exciting, such as your anxious feelings before a presentation helping to keep you sharp and prepared to do your best.

Pay special attention to this next exercise, to make sure that your exposure therapy is not just a misery to be endured but an adventure in discovering your inner thrill-seeker!

EXERCISE Challenging Your Anxiety Sensitivity during Exposure Practice

Before every practice exercise that involves exposure, please do the following, to help you challenge and overcome unhelpful beliefs about your ability to tolerate and thrive while being anxious.

Write down any negative thoughts that predict not being able to do the practice, predict bad things happening during or after the practice, or that reflect your wish to procrastinate, because you fear the anxiety or medical risk the practice might produce.

Then, after your practice, write down what you discovered about your ability to do the exposure practice, to tolerate the physical sensations of anxiety, and to overcome the desire to avoid or curtail the practice. If you're curious and pay attention to what went well, then you'll have the mental health advantage in creating resilience (Babic et. al. 2020). Write down what you did that made this practice such a success.

Here is a sample of what these thoughts might look like, before and after you complete exposure practice.

Exposure	Negative Thoughts Prediction	What I Discovered
Not talking to anyone about my symptoms	*I will have a panic attack and not be able to sleep; I will not be able to get my work done properly because I will be so preoccupied; I will end up crying and be a miserable wreck the following day*	*I got really anxious but after several hours I could focus enough to work out and then get some work done; I didn't have a panic attack, just worried about having one; I fell asleep after a couple of hours and was able to function the next day and not give in to talking to people or texting my doctor*
Not searching for info about skin cancer	*I don't think I can do this without sneaking a peek at WebMD; I won't enjoy going out with my friends if I don't check*	*I was nervous and worried, but able to enjoy the conversation with friends and even laugh a couple of times; I was able to use my phone without searching about skin cancer for the first time in years; I felt better as the night went on and I saw that I could avoid checking WebMD*

Exposure Practice: How You Can Overcome Your Urge to Avoid

Now, we're going to start the process of facing the situations, thoughts, and sensations related to avoidance. Later, in the following chapters, we will deal with using exposure to overcome reassurance-seeking and intolerance of uncertainty.

You can refer to your previous list of negative reinforcers and avoidant thoughts and behaviors for ideas of what to do for your exposure practice. Any activity, thought, or sensation that makes you anxious is good material for exposure practice. (You can add to your lists as you go—many people discover along the way that they are accidentally doing things that they didn't initially realize were unhelpful.)

The easiest way to think about all the things to put on your exposure list is to answer these questions:

1. Are there thoughts, sensations, or situations you have to avoid because of your illness anxiety?

2. Are there words, images, or thoughts about illness that you hate to think about or hear?

3. Are there TV shows, movies, or YouTube videos that you avoid because of illness anxiety?

4. Do you procrastinate or avoid any doctor appointments, tests, or scans?

5. Are you afraid to look at or touch parts of your body, in case you discover something wrong or are reminded of illness or death?

6. Do you avoid getting or looking at your test results?

7. If your anxiety focuses upon the health of someone you love, do you have the same reactions mentioned in numbers one through six, around this person's health?

Planning Your Exposure Practice

Once you have your list, you're ready to plan your exposure practice. The easiest way to design the correct exposure practice is by choosing something that makes you feel anxious and is the opposite of avoiding. That means making a list of things *to do* that face the thoughts, situations, and sensations that you fear.

For example, if you avoid exercising to the point of sweating and losing your breath because you fear having a heart attack or stroke, or accidentally damaging your body, then you will plan to do some physical activities that make you sweat and lose your breath. If you're scared of certain words that remind you of illness and dying, then you need to write and say aloud the words and phrases that scare you. If you avoid watching shows that mention serious illness, cancer, hospice, or chronic disability from illness, then you need to watch these kinds of shows and documentaries. If you're fearful of seeing obituaries about people who have died, then you need to look up and read obituaries. If you avoid or procrastinate scheduling medical appointments or tests, or reading your test results, then you need to schedule some appointments and start reading your test results. If you're afraid to look at certain areas of your body, or to touch them, then you need to start noticing your body and its changes.

EXERCISE Setting Up Exposure Practice for Avoidance

Write down a list of your ideas for how to stop your avoidance and number them.

Your list should look something like this sample list:

1. *Schedule my annual physical and colonoscopy without asking for a later date*
2. *Read these words aloud:* cancer, death, dead, grave, chemotherapy, hospice, untreatable
3. *Watch* Mystery Illness *and medical drama TV shows*
4. *Watch a movie in which a character dies of cancer*

5. *Do a breast self-exam*
6. *Run in place until I sweat and feel hot and dizzy, like something is wrong with my body*
7. *Read obituaries*
8. *Walk through a cemetery and read the tombstones of the newer graves*
9. *Watch YouTube videos of people who are dying of cancer*
10. *Walk through the cancer hospital lobby and sit down in the lobby for ten minutes*
11. *Read medical articles about terminal cancer*

Notice that I didn't ask you to rank your exposures in terms of difficulty. This used to be the way that exposure therapy proceeded, before scientists realized that using the inhibitory learning approach could improve exposure practice.

Instead, we are going to have you pick a system for randomly choosing which exposure practices to do each day, regardless of their difficulty. Here are some suggestions for randomizing your exposure practice so you have an element of surprise.

1. Do even numbers one day and odd numbers the next.
2. Make small paper slips with each exposure written on them, put them in a bowl, and mix them up. Then pick several exposures each day, after placing the previous day's exposures back into the bowl at the end of the day.
3. Let someone else select the numbers for your practice.
4. You could also use three different colored papers: one to highlight numbers 1, 3, 6, another color for 2, 4, 8, and the third color for 5, 7, 9. Then rotate colors every three days.

Each day, I suggest that you commit to doing a certain number of exposures, using your random method of selection. Prior to doing each task, write down your apprehensive thoughts about doing the exposure, and then after, record your evaluation of what it was like to do your practice and how you managed to help yourself through it.

The right number of exposures for you to do is the number that helps you to drop your anxiety level by half and realize that you can do something scary and handle it without avoiding or reassurance-seeking. It should also last long enough or be repeated enough times that it feels less scary, more manageable, or even boring or absurd. For example, you might need to repeat a story about getting seriously ill and dying ten times before it no longer frightens you. You might need to repeat a scary word such as "cancer" two hundred times before it no longer seems scary. You might need to reread an article about someone dying over and over for a half hour before it feels less scary. You might need to go several days or weeks without reassurance-seeking until it feels easier to do.

The obvious exposure practice for avoidance is to face the thoughts, sensations, and situations that make you feel scared, without getting any reassurance by checking, asking, or searching for information or asking someone else's opinion. You want to face the situation until it feels less scary by at least half, or until you find that it no longer makes you anxious. For example, if you fear medical facilities, go sit in the lobby of your nearest medical building or hospital and stay there until you feel 50 percent less anxious or find that it no longer bothers you to be sitting there.

If you want to make your exposure practice efficient and successful, you also need to commit to the following things:

- Do exposure practice every day, or as often as possible.
- Avoid the temptation to undo your exposure practice by thinking avoidance thoughts, i.e. *This is just practice and not the real thing.*
- Avoid reassurance-seeking or checking of any kind for each exposure step you take.

- Ask the people from whom you seek reassurance to kindly remind you that you no longer need their reassurance. You can ask them to say to you, "Looks like you are worrying about illness or dying. Giving you reassurance will only make things worse in the long run. What exposure practice would be most helpful right now?"

Your goal is to conduct daily experiments, to see what really happens when you face your fears—and to compare this with what your anxious mind believed would happen.

Another goal is to inhibit the urge to escape and avoid the exposure practice—thus learning the valuable lesson that you're stronger and more capable during an episode of anxiety than you ever believed possible.

Exposure Practice: Overcoming Fears of Dying, Death, and Disability

My patients often tell me at the beginning of therapy that they hate their imagination, because it makes them think about so many horrible and frightening things. They wish they could turn it off and never have to imagine again anything to do with terrible illnesses, dying, or imagining the dying and deaths of the people they most cherish. Anxious imagination, you may recall, has the power to convince your brain that danger is real and imminent. It can create nightmares and daytime images and thoughts about dying and death that are vivid and difficult to ignore; they reflect your fear of dying or being disabled from serious illness.

Most people who don't have illness anxiety get similar thoughts, but they are able to accept these thoughts and then let go of them because they know that all is well. They realize that what they imagine is not real, and even though they don't like these thoughts, they recognize that they don't have to react to them.

If you want to get over your fear of dying, death, or disability, you'll need to apply exposure practice to your imagination. You can, in effect, inoculate yourself against your fearful imagination, by using exposure practice. In time, you can imagine anything that frightens you, tolerate it, and accept it, without having to do anything in response to the scary thought.

This type of practice in imagination may make you feel teary-eyed or even cry. That is an indication that you're successfully facing your anxious imagination by doing difficult and necessary things. It means that you're doing really well, because you're allowing yourself to experience your anxiety and worst imagined awful future, even though it may initially scare or upset you.

Most of the people I work with quickly lose their strong feeling of sadness and anxiety after the first one or two exposure practices, once they are willing to truly face their fear head-on. You will too. Doing this exposure practice with your anxious imagination will help you learn to ignore the false signal created by your anxiety, to the point where your anxious thoughts no longer feel real and important. Wouldn't that feel great? Cindy's story illustrates what it's like to do this kind of exposure practice.

Cindy's Story

Cindy was a middle-aged woman who repeatedly worried that her partner would die of complications from obesity, diabetes, heart disease, and kidney disease, since her partner was overweight and unable to lose weight. Cindy was a trim, health-conscious person who exercised daily, ate a vegan diet, and meditated to manage stress. Her partner, on the other hand, had never liked exercise, enjoyed foods that Cindy considered unhealthy or even dangerous, and was apparently unconcerned about weighing thirty pounds more than she weighed in her early twenties.

Cindy's partner had recently been prescribed medication for high cholesterol and this triggered Cindy's repeated efforts to get her partner to eat vegan, lose weight, meditate, and adopt the same lifestyle as Cindy. Cindy monitored how much her partner ate, forwarded articles on healthy lifestyle to her partner, and repeatedly worried aloud to her partner, even crying and telling her, "I want you to live a long life with me! Why won't you do something to guarantee that?"

Cindy sought treatment after her partner told her that she could no longer tolerate all the articles, reminders, tears, and worry about dying, and that she felt unloved and heavily criticized by Cindy. Cindy loved her partner and was aghast at her partner's reaction to her concern about her health.

Treatment began with imaginal exposure to her partner's declining health and eventual death. We made a list of different phrases that would scare Cindy, and randomly selected different phrases to practice. Here is an example of some of the phrases: "What if my partner gets heart disease, diabetes, or kidney disease?" "What if my partner dies because I did not warn her and make her change?"

We began by repeatedly saying these scary phrases until they lost their sting and anxiety. Saying these phrases at first made Cindy very anxious and even provoked tears, but she got used to saying them and even got to the point of telling me, "This is boring!"

We progressed to saying other phrases. This too made Cindy teary-eyed, but this time the highest levels of anxiety and tears lasted a shorter time. As Cindy progressed through a series of phrases, she felt scared and sad when she said them, but did not cry as the session progressed. Cindy then practiced saying and writing her list of scary words and phrases every day until it felt 50 percent less scary than when she'd started.

The next time we met, she wrote and read aloud stories about her partner getting ill and tragically dying because Cindy did nothing to help her prevent her death. She marveled that writing this story did not make her break down with tears and anxiety, and told me, "It wasn't as bad as I thought it would be. I can hardly believe that I am writing this kind of story. The worst part was just getting started and knowing that I was going to do this practice."

When you apply exposure practice to your imagination, you should repeat these practices until they no longer make you anxious. It may take you several days or even several weeks of repeating the exposures before they no longer provoke your anxiety. Just as you did with the avoidance exposures, you should write down the thoughts that make you want to avoid your practice, and afterward write down how you managed during the exposures and what you learned about your ability to manage your anxiety.

When I suggest for the first time the practices below, many patients react with horror. They may falsely believe that you should not have to think about dying and death, forgetting that people without illness anxiety are able to hear about other people's severe illnesses, read obituaries, and talk about funerals without undue anxiety. They may grieve and shed tears about the impending death or funeral of someone they love, but they don't avoid thinking or talking about it, or avoid attending wakes or funerals because of anxiety. They are able to accept that the idea of death, dying, and disability is sad, without getting tricked into believing that their worst thoughts are real or useful. Your goal is to become like these non-anxious people, who feel normal sadness and grief without also feeling terrible anxiety.

You may want to put off doing these exercises. If you do, that's a sure sign that these exercises will be very important for helping you obtain a full recovery.

EXERCISE Writing Your Obituary and Eulogy, and Planning Your Funeral*

*If your illness anxiety is about the health of someone else, then do this exercise as though it's that person's death. If you worry about both your health and someone else's, then do these exercises for each person. A worksheet for this exercise is available at http://www.newharbinger.com/49043.

Writing Your Obituary

Write down the obituary that would be posted in the newspaper or social media, mentioning your name, date of death (one month from now), age, cause of death, a few of your accomplishments, surviving family, and the illness-related memorial fund for donations. Once you write it, read it aloud repeatedly until you can do so without tearing up or getting anxious.

Sample Obituary: *Karen Cassiday died on Sunday, June 15, 2019, at the age of 40, after a brief but valiant battle with ovarian cancer. She was a clinical psychologist who loved her work and will be greatly missed by her family, clients, and staff. She is survived by her husband, sister, both parents, two children, three stepchildren, and a dog. Funeral services will be held at Light of Christ Church on Thursday, June 19 at 10 a.m. No flowers please. Memorial donations to the Ovarian Cancer Foundation would be an honor to Karen's life.*

Writing Your Eulogy

Write a speech that someone would give about the tragic loss of your life due to your most feared illness. Mention how there was nothing that could be done and how much everyone will miss you, especially those who love you most. Mention what was significant about your life and what people will fondly remember about you.

Sample Eulogy: *How sad to be gathered here to mourn the loss of someone who was so young and vital. John was my best friend since college, and I can barely believe that he is not going to just walk in the door and grab me in one of his bear hugs and say, "Hey, where's the party?" He was always so cheerful and generous, willing to help me with my studies or to help someone with whatever they needed. When I heard that he got brain cancer, I thought it was a joke. I just couldn't believe that it was him.*

Then, because he was always that guy who did well in life, married the woman of his dreams and had two young boys, I assumed that of course he wouldn't die. I just knew he would beat this. But he didn't.

I am going to miss his bear hugs, his stupid jokes, and his ability to find something good in everyone. Goodbye, John. You're the best friend a guy could ever have."

Planning Your Funeral

Write down all of your instructions for those who survive you, for what should happen at your funeral, burial, and/or in the preparation of your body for burial or cremation. Be sure to cover any religious traditions or spiritual aspects that you want at your funeral. Include the hymns, prayers, or songs that you want, the guest list, the type of casket or urn, the flowers or memorial donations you would like, the type of music or specific songs, the speakers who will eulogize you, and whether or not you want people to share spontaneous memories. Describe the type of artifacts you might want at the wake, meal, or other gathering, such as photographs, trophies, or other mementos. Choose the food that you would like to be served to the funeral guests. Be sure to include details about the burial or scattering of your ashes.

Sample Funeral Instructions: *Call my priest, Father Jones, and he will arrange the funeral service. I want the service to be conducted at Father Jones's church, and for my mother to play the prelude and postlude on the pipe organ. Please have "Be Thou My Vision" sung as one of the hymns and my family can pick the other hymns. Please get the cheapest and least ornamented coffin, since I want to be cremated after the funeral service. Don't waste money on urns. Have my parents leave my ashes in some beautiful place in nature that has a view of the mountains. No open casket. Please serve something chocolate at the wake, since chocolate is one of my favorite foods. Have a time of sharing at my wake, in which people can stand up and share their memories of me. Ask my best friend to do the eulogy and remind her to keep it short. Please let my friends and family divide up my belongings amongst themselves, and give the rest to charity. Have my best friend decide who should take care of my dog. Any money left over after medical and hospital expenses are paid should go to the Golden Retriever Rescue Association.*

If you're having doubts about the utility of doing these exercises, I want you to review your list of the ways your illness anxiety disrupts your life. People who don't have illness anxiety can think about their eventual dying, death, or funeral without undo anxiety. They might feel sad when contemplating their own death, but they don't avoid their thoughts or avoid having conversations about these things.

The truth is, whether you're in good health or are dying, learning to live life to fullest in every moment is the most practical and healthy thing you can do. Giving into your illness anxiety robs you of the ability to live fully and develop the comfortable awareness of your inevitable death, or the inevitable death of someone you love.

My cancer support group patients had it right. When life is the most important thing, you must live it well and with gusto. Trying to ignore the reality of human mortality only increases anxiety. Wise people live well because they have full awareness of the fragility of life and therefore live each moment as well as they can.

Let's summarize what you should be doing to use your exposure practice to overcome avoidance and fear of death, dying, and disability. You should be practicing daily (ideally), or as often as possible. You should not "undo" your practice by reverting to quick escapist thoughts. For example, you should not be telling yourself that your practice is not "real."

You should also try to avoid giving yourself reassurance during your exposure practice. For example, you should resist the urge to remind yourself of the last time your Internet search on your real health age told you that you're five years younger than your chronological age. You should not avoid things after your exposure practice for fear that they will make you more anxious.

Finally, you should ask the people to whom you go for reassurance to gently remind you to stop seeking reassurance. You should select your practice items using a system that's random and unpredictable. You should only retire items from your practice list once they become easy to do and provoke no or very low anxiety.

Next, you'll learn how to tackle the problem of reassurance-seeking.

CHAPTER 4

Giving Up Reassurance-Seeking

The most visible symptom of your illness anxiety is probably the way you regularly seek reassurance from others. When you get anxious, you're at high risk of searching for the people who feel the most reassuring—because they have special medical knowledge, they are kind, they are supportive, or you know they have experienced similar symptoms. You go to them because you cannot help yourself, because you want to know for sure that nothing serious is wrong. You want to go to sleep at night knowing that all is well and that there's nothing to worry about.

Getting reassurance from another person might work temporarily, if you only ask one or two questions and they get answered in a way that feels reassuring. You decrease your sense of uncertainty for the moment, at least until your anxiety comes up with a new serious threat to your health.

Trying to get reassurance is like trying to walk across an interpersonal minefield in which the other person has no map. From their perspective, it looks like you're trying to talk about the likelihood of being okay; they probably don't realize that you're really on a mission to dump your anxiety by getting the perfect reply from them. But they have no idea how to give the perfect response, and they logically realize that they cannot promise you that nothing bad will ever happen.

If the person you ask for reassurance is a health care professional, they feel good about helping you by sharing their expertise. They assume that you ask questions with the intention of following their advice. Health care providers assume that other people will follow their good advice, because it's based upon their expertise. When you accidentally keep repeating the same question, or repeatedly ask related questions, it frustrates your health care provider, because they assume that you don't trust their knowledge or expertise. If you ask about additional tests, referrals, or other types of information, they begin to believe not only that you don't trust them, but that you're uncooperative, because they already considered these things and didn't think that they were important to mention. It would be like you giving a friend your special cake recipe that your friend adores and then having them call you up to ask what you thought about adding broccoli, cheese, and anchovies to the cake batter. This is one reason that many health care professionals end up avoiding you by having you speak to other staff, getting short-tempered with you, or even referring you to another doctor or nurse. They come to believe that they cannot effectively help you, even though they may realize that you're anxious. They also can feel frustrated with the amount of time it may take to try and reassure you, because they feel the pressure to see all of their patients in a timely fashion. Your repetitive questions don't fit into the coding system for billing, which is based in part upon the severity of the diagnosis.

I get frequent calls from the health care providers of those who suffer from illness anxiety. They usually say something like this, "I am not able to help this person. I have been telling them for ages to go and get some help for their anxiety. They never trust what I say and always question everything I suggest. Normally I never order all of the tests that I do for this patient, but I have done it just to try and make them stop bothering me with their worry. I have other much sicker patients who need my time and this person can never accept that they are just fine. " Sometimes I hear worse: "I am so glad that they finally are seeing you because now I can discharge them from my practice. Why do they even come to my clinic when all they do is question everything and never believe that the tests are accurate?"

When your health care provider begins to do the following, it usually means that your anxiety has overstepped the bounds of their professional patience:

- They start their time with you by reminding you that they are on a tight schedule.

- They tell you that you already covered that topic.
- They tell you that they are doing their best, giving you their best knowledge, or that there's no other information to be found (normally this is assumed and they don't feel the need to mention it).
- They tell you that they cannot help you and that you need to talk to a therapist about your illness anxiety.
- They interrupt you to tell you that they need to get to the next patient.
- They tell you that they don't want to order a lab/test/referral, but that they will do it in your case to help you feel less anxious.
- They tell you to stop calling/emailing/texting so they can have time for other patients.
- They tell you to save your questions for the next appointment.

The problem with seeking reassurance from friends, family, or romantic partners is that these people are motivated to make you feel good. When they give you reassurance, they want to see that you get less anxious, feel helped, and trust the relationship. Your repeated questions and anxiety may accidentally convince them that you lack trust in them. They may feel unsuccessful at loving you, and hurt that you cannot trust them enough to feel safe and calm in their presence.

They can also feel put upon when you interrupt their recreation, sleep, dinner, or work by asking questions that don't get resolved. They can feel like you don't respect or care about the boundaries of the relationship, because you're willing to disrupt them at the convenience of your anxiety. They are probably willing to be interrupted on rare occasions when a true crisis exists, but your illness worries don't qualify for this exemption of interpersonal boundaries.

They see that you're worried *and* they see that your worry and reassurance-seeking accomplishes nothing. They just don't know what to do to help you. They feel hurt when you say and do things that make it seem as though the time and love you received from them counted for nothing.

Think of it like this. When you listen and give advice and support to a distressed friend, it feels really good when the friend calms down, smiles, and relaxes. What happens when the friend then calls you back the next day and the next and the next with the same amount of distress about the same issue? Don't you start to feel like nothing you did mattered? Don't you begin to wonder about whether or not that friend trusts you, your advice, or your love?

The same is true for your family, friends, and romantic partner. They assume that their words will provide long-lasting comfort. They also feel challenged when you ask the same question again and again, just like health care providers do. They feel as though you didn't bother to listen the first time or that you don't trust them to give you their best answer.

Reassurance-Seeking Behaviors

Let's take a look at the types of things most people with health anxiety do when they are trying to get reassurance from others:

- Ask others to look at marks, moles, skin blemishes, rashes, stool (feces), urine, snot, mucus, sores, lumps, and bumps
- Ask others to look at comparison photos of the area of the body they are concerned about
- Ask others to feel lumps and bumps
- Ask others to tell them they will be okay, that nothing bad will happen
- Scrutinize others' memory for any knowledge of serious symptoms and detail how this is different from what the worrier knows
- Ask what others' doctor/nurse would say about their symptoms

If you step back from your anxiety for a moment, how appealing is it for anyone who is not a health care professional on duty to do the above things? Is this the kind of thing that brings people closer together? Even if the person *is* a health care professional, do you think this is how they want their friendship, marriage, or relationship with you to be conducted?

When I talk to the partners, family, and friends of people who worry about their health, I get a universal response, regardless of their background: "Please get them to stop! I get so resentful and angry, even though I know anxiety is the problem. I don't want to be talking about these things and trying to figure out how to stop their worry."

There's one type of reassurance-seeking relationship that tends not to experience strain when two people with illness anxiety use each other for reassurance-seeking. But the problem with this relationship is that even though you may both enjoy spending lots of time discussing symptoms, doctors' opinions, and sharing information, and may mutually agree that you can never be too careful or do too much research—you accidentally trap one another into a lifestyle of worry about illness.

Often, I see family members doing this for each other, because they both inherited the same tendency to worry about illness. Their family of origin considers reassurance-seeking, avoidance, and worry about illness to be normal. Although this type of reassurance-seeking relationship might feel beneficial, it's maladaptive. Two worriers might be comfortable with one another's worry, but does this make the worrying helpful? Rethink the wisdom of having reassurance-seeking conversations with others who prefer them, and consider how it hurts you both.

Your illness anxiety drives you to spend hours thinking about, talking about, and comparing notes and opinions. It might feel good in the short run, but you pay a high price for these brief moments of reassurance. The problem with reassurance-seeking is that it backfires in the long run, because it's a negative reinforcer for your anxiety. Remember how in Chapter 2, we reviewed how negative reinforcers always increase your anxiety? It's like your anxiety is a toddler screaming for a reassurance cookie. If you give your worry the cookie of reassurance, then you can expect only one outcome: more illness anxiety.

Additionally, reassurance-seeking prevents you from accepting the normal uncertainty of life. As you read this chapter, keep in mind that your reassurance-seeking is an attempt to reduce uncertainty, by trying to get information that lines up for or against the worst-case scenario. But reassurance-seeking actually only guarantees that your worry about illness, death, and dying will get worse.

The Risks of Playing Doctor

There's a good chance that you have developed expert research skills, and you may even be at an expert level of knowledge about the various facets of diseases that alarm you. This might make you feel qualified to engage in even more reassurance-seeking, by emailing various experts to ask their opinion or by challenging the quality of advice given by a licensed health care professional.

RAISE YOUR RESILIENCE: Don't make the mistake of practicing medicine without a license. It doesn't matter how much research you do or how much information you have. You need a health care professional who can diagnose and treat you, without the impairment of illness anxiety. Avoid the temptation to try and improve upon what your health care professional recommends.

Susan's Story

Susan had a dreaded fear of developing cardiovascular disease and dying an early death. She had many relatives who had died early deaths due to heart disease: heart attacks, strokes, and congenital heart failure. She read many medical journals that cardiologists read, followed all the latest research on exercise and nutrition related to heart disease, and eagerly watched medical training videos about diagnosing various types of cardiac anomalies and heart-related illnesses. She taught herself genetics and read research about the genetic risks and familial transmission of heart disease.

When Susan was referred to me, her cardiologist called me and said, "This patient is the healthiest person in my clinic and she refuses to stop making appointments with me. When she comes into my office, she wants to talk about all the latest research and sometimes knows more about it than I do. She keeps wanting me to do unnecessary tests, in case something is wrong or has deteriorated. Susan gets really upset and angry if I don't give in and order a test. I even put her on a week-long heart monitor to try and prove to her that she was perfectly healthy. It backfired. She read the EKG and noticed a few small abnormalities that amounted to nothing in my opinion, but she knew of a study that showed this might be a precursor to some later problem. She actually had studied EKGs and read her own results! She never listens to me and yet she keeps on coming to me. I refuse to see her again until she completes treatment with you."

This doctor was encountering a person whose anxiety had made her falsely believe that acquiring more knowledge would somehow protect her from disease and premature death. When you let your worry about illness, death, or dying drive you to seek information and become an expert, you're making a cardinal mistake: you're practicing medicine without a license.

Avoid Getting Stuck on the Worst-Case Scenario

Your anxious mind tends to focus on the worst-case scenario, without noticing all the other relevant information. In my office, it's not unusual for my patients with health anxiety to come in with large files containing information about illnesses and diseases they have never experienced. I am quite confident that no one else has this degree of medical information in their file cabinet or on their computer or smartphone unless they too have illness anxiety.

In addition, the very presence of your anxiety renders you ineffective at determining which information is useful and applies to you, and which isn't and doesn't. This is why medical professionals are advised to never treat their own families. Anxiety disrupts your ability to accurately sort through information and determine what is useful and what is not. Anxiety makes everything related to your fear seem equally and significantly important. If you happen to also be a health care provider, you're still disqualified from rendering good decisions about your own health when you're under the influence of illness anxiety, because your anxiety distorts your ability to evaluate anxiety-provoking information.

EXERCISE Stop Practicing Medicine Without a License

Please take out your notebook and write down a declaration with the date and your signature that goes something like this. You can also download a copy of this contract, one for laypersons and one for medical professionals here: www.newharbinger.com/49043.

Layperson's Contract to Stop Practicing Medicine Without a License

I, (insert your name), *vow to stop practicing medicine without a license, and agree to leave the diagnosis and treatment of my health in the hands of my doctors, nurses, and therapists, without doing any of the following:*

- *Researching their opinions to make sure they are the best*
- *Researching for alternative treatments that might be better*
- *Making sure my health care team knows all the same research that I do*
- *Interrogating my health care team, to make sure they really did give me the best information*
- *Researching my health care team's online reviews, background, or publications*
- *Researching every diagnosis and treatment given to me before being willing to try a recommended treatment*

Signed: (Your Name) *Date:*

Your friends with the same health risk factors you have can probably keep their peace of mind when they encounter the information that scares you. People who are not anxious about their own health don't feel the need to research everything known about various diagnoses or treatments, unless they have tried standard treatments and found them to be ineffective. Non-anxious people wait until standard treatments have failed before they start looking around for more information. They assume that their health care providers are attentive, accurate, and giving them useful information. They wait for something to go wrong before they start wondering about what else they need to know and who else they might need to consult.

Once you have done the exercises in this book, you too can begin trusting the expertise of licensed medical professionals.

RAISE YOUR RESILIENCE for Medical Professionals with Illness Anxiety: Your knowledge is not as helpful as you think. Your anxiety about illness, death, and dying is getting in the way. Let your colleagues use their objective and non-anxious skills to help you navigate your health. Be humble and willing to follow their suggestions without trying to improve upon them. They are much more likely to be accurate than you when it comes to your health.

Breaking Up with WebMD

Another common way to seek reassurance is by going online to conduct digital research. I cannot recall any patient with illness anxiety who didn't get trapped spending hours of time on the Internet, comparing their symptoms with the symptoms of various serious illnesses.

The temptation to seek reassurance by going online is strong. It's incredibly easy to use your smartphone, tablet, or computer to rapidly get an image, a video, or a lot of written information about the thing that worries you. You don't even have to use your fingers —you can just tell your smart speaker to find the information you want. The supply of information is endless, and your searches will be too.

Trying to stop online reassurance-seeking is hard. It's like trying to stop eating sweets when you work in a candy factory. Your search engine has likely figured you out and repeatedly sends more health-related information your way because you have searched for it in the past. Furthermore, it's so easy to sneak a peek on your phone when you know that others will assume you're just texting someone. The problem is that as long as you give in to the urge to get reassurance by having an online "date" with WebMD or any other health-related site, you're setting yourself up for failure. You're getting sucked into a really bad blind date that will leave you anxious, worried, and more confused than you were before you got together. That's what happened to Fiona.

Fiona's Story

Fiona worried about getting melanoma, a serious form of skin cancer, so she would check out online images of melanoma every time she felt a bump or saw a mole or discoloration on her skin. One image was never enough. She would then think, What if my skin just doesn't match this particular image but it might match a different image? *Then she would find more and more images, none of which were exactly like her skin. She would change search engines to check to see if the images on Google, for example, were different from the ones on Yahoo or Bing. She even paid for access to a dermatologist's continuing education forum, which allowed her to check hundreds of images of melanomas. Then Fiona would send images of her skin, side by side with images of known melanomas, and ask her family and friends if they thought the photos looked different or the same.*

She would do all of this throughout her workday, in between work tasks, and while at home. She compared images prior to going to bed and each time she woke up in the middle of the night. It made her boyfriend angry and her friends annoyed. Her sister had blocked Fiona's number and email several times, telling her, "You have a problem. This has got to stop!"

Finally, once Fiona went to a dermatologist to get her skin analyzed, the comparisons would stop. Unfortunately, the cycle would start again the next time she detected a new mole or skin discoloration, and would continue for months.

RAISE YOUR RESILIENCE: I'm sure you have your own story of digital reassurance-seeking. In your journal, write down your reasons for doing it. Then, for a moment, be honest with yourself: Is it helping your anxiety? Or making it worse? Like Fiona and Dan, is it straining your relationships? Write down your experience.

If you want to overcome your illness anxiety, even though it seems like the right thing to do, you're going to have to break up with WebMD and all other health-related sources of information. I will help you do this as we move forward.

For now, begin considering that your health care team are the ones who are supposed to be researching your symptoms and illnesses. If you're sincere about no longer practicing medicine without a license, then you need to let the real experts, whose judgment is not clouded by anxiety, do their job. Rather than seek pointless—and temporary—reassurance, I would much rather you use your digital devices to play games, read news, or contact friends.

Conversations with Your Health Care Team

As I have mentioned earlier in this chapter, your in-person reassurance-seeking can take many forms. Here is a list of typical ways I have seen people like you get stuck when relating to a health care team.

- Contacting the pediatrician every time your child gets sick, and insisting that the pediatrician or nurse check your child's symptoms just to make sure.
- Trying to engage nurses and doctors in conversations and asking them to tell you that nothing serious is going on, even though they already announced that your child has an easily treatable common cold, flu, or viral illness.

- Asking the nurse and doctor how many other kids they have seen with the same symptoms, to make sure that it really is a common illness that is going around and not something serious.
- Quizzing other parents in the doctor's lobby about their kids' symptoms, to make sure that your kid is not unlike everyone else's, and then asking the receptionist if lots of other patients have had the same symptoms and if they are getting better.
- Texting and posting on social media about your child's minor illness, to see if others will affirm that your child will be okay.
- Making your partner, family, and friends a part of your health care team by, for example, asking your partner to examine a spot, rash, mole or other skin irritation to see if it looks cancerous. Then polling friends to see if they have any spots, rashes, or discolorations like yours and whether or not it was diagnosed as skin cancer.
- Sending symptoms or photos to the doctor or specialist and trying to get their opinion on whether or not you should go in for an in-person appointment.
- Interrogating your doctor about how they know it's not a serious problem, and repeatedly asking for tests when the doctor didn't initially order one, just to make sure that nothing is wrong. Then asking all the clinic staff if they have seen other patients with the same symptoms and what their diagnosis was.
- Repeatedly calling in to after-hours call-in lines or virtual consultations about your health worries.
- Your health care provider's staff recognizes you by voice and may have made jokes about needing to issue frequent flyer care.
- You frequently have the feeling of not being able to wait to call a doctor, nurse, or therapist, and have sat waiting for the clinic or help line to open.

If you identify with even a few of these things, then you're undoubtably getting stuck in a reassurance-seeking relationship with your health care team. Also, if, like many of my patients with illness anxiety, you choose your doctors solely on the basis of getting constant access to someone you can talk to about your worries, then you have a problem.

Conversations with health professionals *can* be helpful. But here's the difference: reassurance-seeking conversations focus on the negative and wanting to make sure nothing is wrong. When your doctor tells you that you're okay, you tend to want to ask, "Are you sure?" even though you just got good news.

Reassurance-seeking conversations also focused on getting absolute certainty when none can be had. For example, you want to hear the doctor not only say that you don't have cancer, but that you'll never get cancer. Your questions are repetitive and directed toward getting a black-and-white ruling, when no test or diagnosis can be perfect and permanent for your lifespan.

Typical reassurance-seeking conversations tend to start off with these questions. Have you heard yourself asking any of them?

- "Have you ever heard of anything like this?"
- "Have you ever known someone who had symptoms like these?"
- "Are you sure I, or someone I love, is okay?"
- "Are you sure it's not something serious?"
- "Are you sure I, or they, will get better?"
- "Have you ever heard of someone who had this ending up with cancer/dying/disabled?"
- "What if this doesn't get better?"
- "Shouldn't I get a test to make sure that I, or someone I love, am okay?"
- "Are you sure that these test results are right?"
- "Shouldn't I get another test?"

- "What is the false-negative rate on this test?"
- "Is there a better or more definitive test for this?"
- "Have you ever seen someone with this not do well?"

These questions all lead in one direction: toward your health care provider being pushed to mention some rare case of an exception to the rule that then triggers all your inner alarm bells. You accidentally end up even more anxious than when you started, without getting what your fear really craves: absolute certainty that nothing bad will happen.

Since none of us can escape the fact that we will someday die and likely experience various illnesses during our lifetime, anyone who wants to reassure you gets stuck between the logical problem of knowing both that you're okay and also that you'll likely someday experience disease, dying, and death. Whether they are a doctor, friend, or family member, they get stuck in a no-win situation of wanting to make you feel better but knowing the facts of life.

This is why the people who are on the receiving end of your reassurance-seeking can get so irritated with you. They see that their efforts to help are only making things worse, and they lack the clinical training to properly address the true source of your anxiety.

As we'll explore in depth in the next chapter, your real enemy is your intolerance of uncertainty.

Dan's Story

Dan would go to the Internet every time his children got any rash, cough, or headache, and type in the symptoms to see which serious diseases these symptoms might match.

If he came up with nothing, he would then make sure his children were healthy by going to other medical websites of various renowned medical institutions. If some of the symptoms overlapped with serious diseases—for example, headache can be a symptom of brain cancer, stroke, aneurysms, encephalitis, and more—then he would begin exhaustive research into each of the serious diseases that contained the symptom his child experienced.

Dan would lose sleep while staying up to do this. He tried to hide his online reassurance-seeking from his wife by sneaking it in during his workday, and so he could try to refrain from learning about upsetting symptoms of serious illnesses at home. It was so bad that his wife would get angry when she saw him on his phone or laptop for any extended period of time. She would assume he was doing online reassurance-seeking and accuse him of having an affair with his laptop or phone, because he was no longer in bed to cuddle her at bedtime.

Breaking the Reassurance-Seeking Habit

Breaking the reassurance-seeking habit may be a challenge, but it's achievable and necessary for your recovery. To do so, you'll use exposure therapy, combined with response prevention. The exposure part will be simply allowing yourself to feel worry about illness, dying, or death. The response prevention part will entail refusing to get reassurance, by avoiding online searches about medical conditions and treatments, conversations about your illness worries, and medical consultations and tests that your doctor did not recommend.

I don't suggest setting unrealistic goals of complete abstinence, which is a common mistake. You're bound to just get discouraged when you slip and indulge in reassurance-seeking. It's much more effective to set goals that are smaller, more specific, and easier to attain. The easiest way to do this is to set goals that allow you to focus upon specific situations you can master, one at a time. After you master one situation, then you can move to the next situation, and gradually add each accomplishment as you learn to successfully avoid giving in to the urge to seek reassurance.

You're more likely to succeed when you divide your goals for stopping reassurance-seeking into the people, situations, and websites that you tend to seek when anxious.

Danielle's Story

Danielle discovered that she could succeed when we worked in small daily steps to eliminate seeking reassurance online. First, Danielle deleted medical websites and bookmarks from all of her medical devices, and set up certain time periods each day when she deliberately would not go online to look at medical information, starting with ten-minute increments.

Once she was able to go thirty minutes without visiting medical websites, she increased the time by ten minutes every five days, until she could go several hours without visiting medical websites. She kept track of the number of minutes she was successful at avoiding online medical searches every day, to help remind her of her successes. This motivated her to keep going, because it showed her the daily and cumulative progress she had made.

Once she could go three hours without seeking reassurance online, she did imaginal exposure to the illnesses she dreaded, such as terminal cancer, all the while avoiding visiting medical websites. She put up sticky notes around her house to remind her to think about cancer. Then she set the goal of no online reassurance-seeking for a half-day, while increasing the time every few days by thirty-minutes increments, until she could go all day without any online reassurance-seeking, while simultaneously bringing to mind her upsetting thoughts about cancer and dying.

Once Danielle achieved this milestone, she began working on eliminating reassurance-seeking conversations with the people she went to for reassurance, choosing one person at a time to stop talking to about her illness worries. Next, she asked these same people to stop giving her reassurance, no matter how much she made excuses or begged.

Her last step, the most difficult one, was to allow me to talk to her doctor and staff about no longer giving her reassurance. Instead, I asked them to simply tell her, "It looks like your anxiety is really bothering you. I don't want to make it worse by accidentally giving you reassurance. How about you talk about this with your therapist and come back to me if she says it's okay for us to talk about this?"

Stopping your reassurance-seeking is very important and is often the major stumbling ground for many who worry. Your ability to succeed will depend on your willingness to stop reassurance-seeking and to embrace the idea that you no longer need to make sure that nothing bad is happening. That means wholeheartedly believing that your biggest problem is your anxiety about illness, dying, and death, as opposed to whether or not you, or someone you love, is seriously ill or dying.

RAISE YOUR RESILIENCE: Most people need to enlist the help of others to fully overcome reassurance-seeking. Be willing to ask for help. Write down in your journal or notebook names of people you can contact who will encourage you to follow through with stopping reassurance-seeking behavior. Be willing to ask people to stop giving you reassurance, even when you seem really anxious.

Reassurance-Seeking Is a Dangerous Thing

Another factor to consider is that reassurance-seeking is something that you cannot do a little bit of and then have no consequences. It's the anxiety equivalent of trying to just do a little bit of crack cocaine (a drug considered to be one of the most powerful drugs to create an instant craving) and then being disappointed by the immediate craving for the next dose of crack cocaine.

Once you give up reassurance-seeking, you have to make the commitment to be resolute, with no turning back. This usually requires requesting the help of others. Here are some examples of beneficial ways of requesting help:

- Asking someone to stop giving you reassurance and giving them something else to say that is genuinely helpful, such as "Looks like you're really anxious. I don't want to make things worse by giving you reassurance. Let's change the topic."

- Telling your supportive friends that you're trying to reduce reassurance-seeking and need their help to point out when you slip into reassurance-seeking mode.
- Telling your doctor that you get anxious about your health and that your anxiety makes you seek their reassurance. Tell them that you need their help to not get stuck in repetitive anxious questioning.
- Asking your supportive friends and family to help you do other things besides researching medical information.

David's Story

Here is another example of how to decrease online reassurance-seeking. David had certain websites that he liked to go to for information about cancer. He had done a lot of research to determine which websites had the best and the latest information, and preferred to go to the ones that were affiliated with the top cancer researchers.

David agreed to start decreasing his online reassurance-seeking by stopping visits to the least important website for a week at a time. The following week, he agreed to eliminate the next website that was least important, while continuing to avoid the first website, and so forth, until he was no longer visiting any websites.

This worked well for David, since he had five sites that he felt were reliable and ignored other websites. He also texted me each day to report his successes, to help him mark his progress and maintain accountability. He also stopped all of his subscriptions to cancer research updates and cancer research listservs. I reminded him throughout that although these various sites were good sources of information about cancer, he didn't need to read them until he was diagnosed with cancer.

EXERCISE Escaping the Trap of Reassurance-Seeking

So, now it's your turn to set some goals for breaking up with your reassurance-seeking. You are going to write down a list of the people, websites, news feeds, or other online domains you visit for the purpose of seeking reassurance. Take out your journal or notebook and make a list like the one below. Next to each type of reassurance-seeking you engage in, write down your first step(s) toward breaking this particular habit. You can also download worksheets to help you with these two exercises here: www.newharbinger.com/49043.

Your list will look something like this:

Reassurance-Seeking	Ways to Wean Myself
Going to WebMD and famous university medical websites for info on cancer	*Start with only doing this 3 times/day* *1/day, then 1/every other day, etc.*
Reading research on cancer prevention and cancer cures	*Set a date to stop doing this*
Reading about carcinogens (cancer-causing agents)	*Cancel my newsletters about this* *Stop talking to the health food store owner and clerks about the newest info* *Stop taking home the free magazines from the health food stores*
Filling out Internet quizzes on my cancer risk	*Read books when I'm alone instead of going on my tablet*
Interrogating friends and family about the cause of their cancer	*Think of other things to talk to cancer survivors about*

Reassurance-Seeking	Ways to Wean Myself
Sending articles about cancer to my friends and family to see if they think I should do anything	*Send funny videos and cartoons instead* *Ask them to stop sending me cancer-related stuff*
Reading about cancer survivors	*Stop subscriptions to cancer survivors newsletters, blogs, and podcasts*
Asking the receptionist, nurses, and doctor if they think I'm okay	*Ask them about themselves* *Only ask my doctor 1) what she/he thinks is the problem and 2) what I should do*
Researching the meaning of my lab tests	*Just let the doctor or nurse explain it* *Stop trying to find if they missed something*
Getting doctor appointments and tests to make sure I'm okay	*Only make doctor appointments when I'm sick or for my annual physical*
Buying over-the-counter blood and urine tests to make sure I'm okay	*Only go to the drive-through window at the pharmacy so I'm not tempted to pick up a new test to self-administer*
Checking my blood pressure to make sure it's not too high	*Avoid the part of the store with the check-your-blood-pressure station* *Give away my blood pressure cuff to someone who has high blood pressure*

Here are some helpful reminders from Chapter 2 that will make it easier to do your exposure practice to stopping reassurance-seeking.

Write down your negative expectations about what it will be like to do the exposure practice of going without reassurance when you're worried about illness. This helps get you clear about the anxious thinking that you're going to undermine with your practice.

Construct your list of possible exposure practices for giving up reassurance-seeking. Give each item a number so you can use a method of random selection for your practice. This will prevent your anxiety from selecting which items to practice.

Practice doing the item you selected until your anxiety drops by at least half, or until you feel comfortable enough that you're no longer at risk for giving in and seeking reassurance. What is really important is to keep doing your exposure practice without giving in. Giving in to the urge to get reassurance undermines your exposure and reinforces your worry. It will take courage, which is your ability to do things when you're afraid. The more you practice doing things that provoke your illness anxiety without seeking reassurance, the more courageous and anxiety-free you'll become.

Remind yourself that the most important thing that you're practicing is how to feel worried and anxious without giving in to the urge to seek reassurance. Your worry will try to misdirect you into believing that inadequate health care, tragic illness, or lack of specialists are the problem instead of your anxiety about illness. Remember, your enemy is your illness anxiety, not actual illness or fate.

If you can, practice every day. This will increase your confidence in your ability to face and manage your anxiety without reassurance-seeking. It will also help your anxiety and worry to decrease.

Finally, evaluate and reflect on how you managed your anxiety during your exposure practice. Was it as difficult as you thought? Did your anxiety last as long as you expected? What did you do that helped you succeed at not giving in to your anxiety? What did you learn that will help you do the next practice?

If you get anxious about someone else's health and have trouble with reassurance-seeking, then you'll want to hear the story of Anna's recovery.

Anna's Story

Anna was a mother who worried about the health of her children. She would call the pediatrician every week during the call-in hour when the pediatrician would answer any parents' questions or concerns. She talked almost daily with her mother and a close friend about the symptoms her children experienced. She would also take repeated temperature readings from multiple thermometers on multiple parts of her children's bodies, any time they appeared ill.

Anna began her recovery by first asking her mother and her friend to tell her if she was asking too many questions about her children's health. Once Anna was able to forego getting reassurance from her mother and friend for a full week, she decided to stop talking to her friend about health concerns, and asked her friend to remind her to not ask for reassurance. Once she succeeded at this, she asked her mother to stop giving her reassurance. She told both of these people that she wanted to keep talking with them, just not about her children's health. This was a challenge for all of them, because her children's health had become the chief topic of conversation. She developed several open-ended questions to ask, to steer the conversation in a productive direction, such as "What was the funniest thing that happened at work today?" or "Where would you like to take a vacation?"

Anna's most difficult challenge was giving up the weekly call-in hour with her pediatrician, because talking to the pediatrician felt like her safety net, in case something was seriously wrong with her children. She used exposure practice to imagine all of her worst fears about what would happen if she failed to consult the pediatrician, such as her children dying tragic deaths that could have been prevented by early intervention if only had she called the doctor in time.

Once she could tolerate the thought of the tragic deaths of her children, she agreed to call her pediatrician only once every other week for a month. Once she met that goal, she stopped calling the pediatrician unless one of her children had any of the symptoms that the American Academy of Pediatrics listed as a reason to call the doctor. She also began practicing taking only one temperature reading from one body site within one hour, and only if one of her children was complaining of actual symptoms of fever. She also agreed to stop feeling her children's foreheads to verify their health status, and began to use just one thermometer for all temperature readings.

RAISE YOUR RESILIENCE: Your anxiety and awareness of uncertainty will increase during the early stages of your exposure practice. This is a sign that you're doing the right practice—because it's making you uncomfortable. This is a sign of success and courage! Take the time to acknowledge your progress and bravery in your journal or notebook. This is your opportunity to push back against illness anxiety.

In the next chapter, we will talk about ways to improve your ability to directly challenge your intolerance of uncertainty. In the meantime, know that many other people just like you have been successful in stopping their reassurance-seeking and you will be too, if you keep at it. Be persistent and patient as you move past this obstacle in your quest for an illness anxiety–free life. I promise it's worth all of your effort!

CHAPTER 5

Higher Tolerance of Uncertainty Can Decrease Your Anxiety

At the heart of illness anxiety is a desire for certainty about your health, or the health of someone you love. This may sound obvious and not worth mentioning, since you may assume that everyone feels the same—don't we all want to make sure we live a long, healthy life and experience a relatively painless death? The truth, however, is that the majority of people are quite comfortable with not knowing when and how they will get ill, when they will die, or how they will die.

Like you, non-worriers are aware that things could go tragically wrong with their own, or their loved one's health. But they don't worry about it until they are diagnosed with a serious or terminal illness. Non-worriers don't downplay how upsetting it would be if they were to succumb to a serious illness or become terminally ill. They are able to not get upset about the possibility ahead of time, since they know they cannot control what the future brings.

They also don't believe they are particularly unfortunate should they, or someone they love, become seriously or terminally ill. They live by this idea: "Why not me? Why not someone I love? I want to enjoy the present moment, because worrying won't make it easier if something terrible happens."

These thoughts may seem strange to you, because they express an acceptance of risk and uncertainty that is hard to imagine when you're fraught with illness anxiety. People who don't worry about their health express an awareness that the only moment we can influence is the present moment. They recognize that we cannot control the future and they understand that worry confers no advantage upon the worrier. "Do the best you can with what you have" might be their motto.

> **RAISE YOUR RESILIENCE:** In your journal, write down what might happen if you took this practical and reasonable approach to your health. Wouldn't it feel less anxiety-provoking to spend most of your mental and emotional energy making the most of each day, without fearing what will happen in the future? Write about what that would feel like.

Maximizers Versus Satisficers

This practical and clear-eyed way of taking advantage of the good that is available is what scientists call *satisficing* (Schwartz et al. 2020). It starts with giving up your pursuit of the best possible guarantee that nothing bad can happen to your health. Satisficing is what happens when you're content with getting enough of what you want, without having to make it perfect. People who are satisficers tend to be content with their decisions and their lives, and feel happy with their current situation.

Maximizers, on the other hand, are people who are always trying to make sure that things are the best. They want their decisions, possessions, relationships, jobs, and hobbies to be the best they can be. They assume that there must always be a better way to do things, but this leads them into misery, instead of guaranteeing them a better life.

If you're a maximizer, you take an accidentally narrow and inflexible approach to life, by creating an idea of how things should be that doesn't account for normal variation and mistakes. Any deviation from your mental image of the right thing feels very wrong—catastrophically wrong. Maximizing is strongly correlated with perfectionism, anxiety, depression, and elevated risk for suicide (Smith et al. 2018). Maximizers are much more likely to experience regret about their decisions, whether it's the purchase of a new phone, a consultation with a particular doctor, or the choice of which vaccine to take. They are also less likely to feel happy, because there's no human way to guarantee that you have done the best, gotten the best information, or consulted with the best doctors. This is the opposite of how many people who are not anxious about their health function.

When it comes to their health, maximizers feel that it's only appropriate to talk to the very best doctor, get the very best test, or visit the very best hospital. If you're a maximizer, you'll compare and contrast all the features of your doctors or treatment, and spends hours comparing them to other experts and doing extensive research on side effects, failure rates, patient reviews, professional background, etc. You'll then accidentally make any decision about your health care a long, laborious process, in your attempt to eliminate uncertainty by making the very best decisions.

Contrast this with satisfiers, who tend to be happy, content, and free from anxiety and depression. When they are trying to get information, or make a decision about their health care, once they find the first thing that is useful, they stop searching for more information. They make decisions about their health care easily, because as soon as they see that something or someone addresses a need or provides an answer, they accept that choice or answer and stop searching. If you're a satisfier, you don't concern yourself with trying to find the best test, doctor, or hospital. You focus on what is the easiest way to get the job done.

Do you see the difference between these two opposing ways of approaching decisions about your health care, and how it can have such a profound effect? If you're like the patients I see, then you're always in a fruitless quest for the best medical opinion, the best treatment, the best diagnosis, or the best odds of preventing a serious illness. This tendency to maximize interacts with your intolerance of uncertainty in a vicious way. It fools you into believing that you can get rid of uncertainty by making sure that anything you do related to health care is the very best, which in turn feels like it lowers the odds of something bad happening.

Reasons to Let Go of Maximizing

You might feel like arguing with me at this point. This is how most of my patients feel when I first suggest letting go of the pressure to find the best that medicine has to offer. You're likely asking yourself, "Aren't people more likely to get excellent care if they see the best person in the field?" But there's no evidence to support this idea. Here are some perspectives to consider as you learn to address your anxiety.

Specialists Are Not Required

Let's take the example of developed countries that have socialized medicine, such as Great Britain, France, Canada, or Norway. Their care is mediated by general practitioners, as opposed to specialists. What we see is that people living in these countries have a longer lifespan and experience fewer lifestyle-related illnesses. People in these countries see specialists only when their general practitioner sees the need, when something unusual or serious occurs that doesn't respond to the recommended first-line treatments.

The population statistics don't lie. What we see in these countries is that people use more preventive care and have easier access to health care providers—in general and specialist care—when they need it. This proves the point that we need good health care, not specialist health care.

Your Health Providers Do Care

Your typical pediatrician, internist, family practice doctor, nurse, or nurse practitioner is highly motivated and highly trained to distinguish benign symptoms from significant ones. They see dozens of people every day and have much more experience than you might realize. They also want to be the person who helps you, who improves your health, and who detects things that are significant. This is in contrast to the frequently voiced worry that "My doctor is being sloppy, lazy, or doesn't really care about my health as much as I do."

Their internal professional motivation is strongly in your favor, even when they might be tired or working late or responding to an emergency. They take great pride in protecting your health and most do this job because they love it.

The amount of effort they had to expend to become your health care provider weeded out people who were not truly passionate about going into health care. When you realize this, it's easy to see that your health care provider is on your side all of the time, even when they don't agree with you. You have every reason to trust their motivation, their skill, and their dedication to your health care.

RAISE YOUR RESILIENCE: When you accept that there's no such thing as the best health care or the best doctor or the best information, you make it easier to recover from your illness anxiety. You just need information that is useful and a medical team that can get the job done.

The Treatment Reality for Common Illnesses

The assumption that only the best will do puts you at odds with the reality of how common illnesses are treated. Unless you really do have a rare condition that only an expert understands, what you need is a health care team that is competent and qualified to diagnose and treat your overall health. Since the majority of your health concerns involve common conditions, a licensed family doctor, pediatrician, general practitioner, or internist is all that is required. They address multiple examples of your type of health concerns every day and, if they are licensed, meet the standard of being experienced and knowledgeable. They know when to refer patients to specialists because of limitations in their training and experience. No medical professional wants to be one who overlooks something serious!

Your Wise Inner Voice Is Not Anxious

When you always defer to the quest for the best, you undermine your ability to trust your own healthy—as in, non-anxious—judgment. You also undermine your ability to trust the good judgment of your health care team. If you take a maximizer's approach to your health care, you increase the risk of falling prey to worries such as, "What if my doctor is not aware of the latest research? Shouldn't I get a second opinion to make sure I'm okay? Maybe I should have someone else read my test results?"

Each time you ignore your own good judgment that realizes nothing is wrong, you weaken your ability to hear and respond to this wise inner voice. You begin to believe that you cannot trust and believe in the idea that all is well. You convince yourself that only a qualified expert can decide whether or not you're okay. You increase the odds of reassurance-seeking, "just to make sure." In short, you guarantee that the misery of illness anxiety becomes imbedded in your life, while actually gaining nothing when it comes to better health or reduced anxiety.

RAISE YOUR RESILIENCE: Ignoring the urge to get a second opinion, find a more expert doctor, or visit a specialist will increase your ability to trust your non-anxious judgment. Journal about what it would feel like to trust your wise inner voice. Try to imagine how much less overwhelmed you would be if you trusted the opinion of your health care team.the first time around. Picture the extra time and the freedom from the burden of research and consultation you would feel. Imagine what it would be like to trust your own opinion and your doctor's without feeling the need to second-guess.

Your recovery will depend on you learning to listen to your healthy, non-anxious voice when it tells you, "This is just your anxiety and nothing to worry about." It will become important to give up the search for the best in medical care, in an effort to reduce the long-term discomfort you feel. Searching for the very best information will not change the fact that you're like everyone else who lives in a human body that is subject to illness and eventually death. Perfect preventive care and perfect health care will not protect you from your body's aging and eventual death.

It's true that good health habits will improve the quality of your health and increase the likelihood that you'll live longer, with less disability, but it's never a guarantee. You're going to have to decide to live well in the imperfect present moment, by accepting that your worry accomplishes nothing toward better health or better health care.

The Fundamental Facts of Human Living and Dying

You likely believe that serious illness, dying, and death are tragic, unfair events—especially when they occur before someone is at the end of a long, well-lived life. Perhaps you subscribe to the ideas that "People who live well should be rewarded by long and happy lives and have children who live long and happy lives," or that "Nothing bad should happen to children, teens, and adults until they live a very long life." While you might never have clearly stated these two ideas aloud to yourself, if you're honest, it's highly likely that you act and talk as though these two ideas are true.

For example, at a funeral for someone who died before age forty, you might say things like, "This is so unfair. She was only thirty-eight. It seems like only the good die young." Or do you secretly think things like this when you hear of a young person getting a serious chronic illness: "Why does this have to happen to someone who is so good and so innocent? Why doesn't this happen to bad people, or people who murder others?"

These thoughts are understandable. Our culture promotes the idea that virtuous people will be rewarded, and evil people will suffer torment. Unfortunately, a quick survey of who gets ill or experiences tragedy reveals that it can happen to anyone at any time, and doesn't seem to correlate with virtue or character.

Almost all of my patients subscribe to these ideas without realizing it until we discuss it in treatment. Consider the alternative, more helpful way to think in response to sad or tragic news: "This is so sad and difficult. I wish you didn't have to go through this and I wish that there was something I can do." That acknowledges the other person's pain, while accepting the circumstances without getting stuck in existential blame.

In treatment, we're seeking less resistance to the following facts of life:

- Tragedy cannot be prevented by moral living, being wealthy, or avoiding all carcinogens.
- There's a good chance that your family, and those you know, have experienced serious illness, disability, cancer, early death, automobile accidents, war, and illness or death.
- It's true that if you're a person of color, live in poverty, or live in a war-torn area, then you're at risk of experiencing overall worse health, earlier death, and serious injury, but no more than your neighbors who share your circumstances.
- Part of being human means living in a body that is vulnerable to germs, toxic substances, accidents, and the passing of time.
- All humans will eventually die. However, no human gets to know the exact hour of their death or the manner in which they will die, until it's upon them. You might not have thought about your death in this manner, but it's something that we all must do, just as we all must be born into this world.
- Just as we didn't get to choose the way we were born into this world, we don't get to choose the manner in which we leave it. These are two facts that we all share, no matter who we are.
- We have no way of knowing if we, or someone we love, will live a short or a long life.
- We have no way of knowing if we, or someone we love, will be subject to random tragedy.

RAISE YOUR RESILIENCE: It's easier to overcome your intolerance of uncertainty when you accept that illness, dying, and death are universal. Take some time to pause and think how all of humankind shares in these experiences of human suffering, and to realize that you're not alone in this. Sometimes just thinking about the universality of something is enough to make us feel less alone, and more connected to our fellow humans.

Why Accepting These Truths Is Helpful

When you hear these existential truths, you can begin to understand that illness, dying, and death are not unfair events, but instead are profound commonalities that we share with all people. You realize that the misfortunes of illness and dying are experiences of suffering that are universal. This counters your unhelpful belief that illness is something unfair or uniquely dealt out by a punishing god. It also may help you begin to work on accepting the idea that being human means living with and enduring the suffering of a human body that breaks down with illness, dying, and eventually death.

I volunteered in the department of psychiatry and behavioral health in Bhutan, a small country in the Himalayas that is the only officially Buddhist country in the world. Everyone there is taught from the cradle that life involves both profound suffering and great joy.

Bhutan's value system is the opposite of ours in the West, which espouses the idea that good only comes to those who earn it or deserve it, and that success means living a life that avoids suffering. People in the West often act as though it's their right to avoid suffering, because they did the right things, sought the right advice, and lived good lives. But as a result of their acceptance of suffering, the Bhutanese learn to fully enjoy the beauty of the moment and to cultivate the virtues of compassion, forgiveness, generosity, tolerance, humility, full awareness of self and others, and gratitude for any good that comes their way.

Bhutan is also a country with limited resources and a simple lifestyle. The Bhutanese approach life with a gentle acceptance of what it means to be human in a world in which uncertainty is an everyday occurrence. Living in Bhutan for three months brought into sharp contrast the clash between the Western maximizing, avoiding suffering, and controlling the future way of thinking. People in Bhutan still get anxiety, but their intolerance of uncertainty is much easier to manage, due to their cultural recognition of the suffering inherent in the human condition. They already know that any moment of peace, good health and happiness are worth savoring because dying and death are around the corner.

Acceptance of the universal suffering of illness, dying, and death makes it easier to deal with your illness anxiety in the following three ways:

1. You flip the idea of avoiding random tragedy on its head, by agreeing with the idea that suffering happens just because you're human. This takes away the pressure to gets things perfectly right in order to guarantee that nothing bad happens.

2. It also puts something very important into perspective. Because suffering and death are inevitable, the very best way to live is to enjoy the present moment and to be fully emotionally available for every bit of good you experience each day. You realize that fun, joy, and being healthy and alive are special moments worth relishing and celebrating.

You begin to feel grateful for every healthy and pleasant moment you, or the ones you love, have—because you know that someday you'll die. It becomes easier to shift your perspective from profound worry into profound gratitude that right now, you're alive and able to read this book.

Your goal is to refocus on what is good in the present moment, instead of what might happen in the future, which you'll never be able to control.

You can acknowledge that you're at no greater, nor lesser, risk for health tragedy than anyone else, no matter what your worry might say.

If others can learn to accept the uncertainty of being a human, then you can too. If others can learn to suffer well, by celebrating and paying attention to the joys and blessings of each moment of life, then you can too. If others can learn to suffer well when they are sick and take pleasure in the little things, then you can too. You can learn to take the attitude that my oncology support group patients took: "I'm going to do the best that I can to enjoy life now, because I'm not dead yet!"

Dare to switch your belief system from one that favors doing things the "best" way and doing things to eliminate uncertainty. Think about the benefits of deciding to accept the universal experience of being a human who is born, suffers, and dies, without ever knowing when or why it will happen. Remind yourself that you're not alone and that every human who has ever lived has had to deal with this truth of their uncertain existence. Recognize that the best response to this truth is to savor and enjoy every moment of good health, good feelings, good experiences, and good relationships that life brings. Realize that the all the little moments of love—such as sharing a good hug, cuddling with your partner, viewing a beautiful sunrise, hearing a magical moment in a musical performance, smelling the sweet, intoxicating fragrance of flowers—are all precious gifts that are your privilege to embrace, if only you decide to savor them and perceive the beauty of these ordinary moments.

Your entire life is a gift, and I suggest that you receive it as such, instead of wasting precious time worrying about the imagined awful future.

Uncertainty in All Areas of Life

Intolerance of uncertainty often extends to other areas of your life, including the following. You might:

- Dislike surprises, want to know everything ahead of time, and not want to wait to learn news, such as the gender of an unborn baby, the outcome of a placement exam, or what happened to your job application.

- Find not knowing something to be very uncomfortable. You may track the location of your child or partner to make sure they are safe, or ask friends and family to call or text as soon as they arrive—even calling them before they arrive to remind them to call you.
- Be afraid of getting lost when you travel to new places, so you always want a complete itinerary for every trip and vacation, because not having one makes you feel uncomfortable.

If you do these kinds of things to manage your fear of uncertainty, then you should also plan to do exposure practice to get rid of your intolerance of uncertainty, for the sake of making it easier to maintain your recovery from your illness anxiety. Your uncertainty exposure practice should be done in the same manner as described in Chapter 4. You can download a worksheet here: www.newharbinger.com/49043.

Here are the steps you should take:

- You'll need to list uncertain situations that trigger your anxiety, such as those mentioned above.
- Then use a random method to select a situation to practice, only in this case instead of avoiding getting reassurance, *you're going to avoid finding out or planning out ahead of time how things will go.*
- Take the time to identify your negative expectations about how you'll handle your anxiety and the situation.
- List the worst thing that could happen when you have uncertainty. For example, "I will not be able to enjoy vacation if I don't plan out every day."
- Practice being in the state of uncertainty and not knowing for sure. Do this without getting any additional information. This is an all-or-nothing type of exposure, so no cheating by finding out ahead of time or giving in to the urge to plan or prepare.

- Evaluate how you handled the exposure and reflect upon your negative predictions and what really happened. Take stock of what you did that made your experience successful and plan to repeat that with the next practice.

Throughout your journey with the exposure practices in this book, deliberately embrace the uncertainty of your life—because you now realize that your uncertainty about life is normal, universal, and inevitable. You'll feel the sharp contrast to the tragic, personalized, and punishing way your anxiety wants to frame things. This is the way my oncology support group members viewed their lives and it served them well in turning away from worry about what was to come, when they knew they could not change the course of their disease.

When you stop making tragedy and suffering personal and punishing, you can instead welcome the awareness that a certain amount of tragedy and suffering is random and can occur to anyone, regardless of their resources or circumstances. Knowing that, you'll let go of the idea that suffering is unfair, and instead celebrate the fact that every human also has the opportunity to enjoy the good moments that occur each day, because they are blessings in the midst of universal human suffering.

CHAPTER 6

Dealing with Real Health Risks

People who thrive view the stressors in their lives as challenges to be met, offering opportunities for growth or insight that are impossible to obtain any other way. When my sister was dying of cancer, she exemplified this attitude and told me, "I never would have learned how many wonderful people are out there had it not been for cancer. I never would have gotten over my shyness either! I feel so blessed that I learned these things while I'm still alive." Anxiety is not synonymous with having a serious illness.

If you do have health conditions that are chronic, serious, and require medical intervention—even a terminal illnesses, such as cancer, end-stage renal disease, or end-stage lung disease—then you might fear that treatment for illness anxiety runs counter to treatment for your health problem. You may also be concerned that decreasing your conversations with your health care team, or decreasing research for treatments and cures, puts you at risk for a shorter or more painful life. This assumption is incorrect.

The goal of successful treatment for illness anxiety is to help you learn how to interact with your health care team effectively, so you can enjoy your life without spending unnecessary time in your head, living in an awful imagined future of illness, dying, and death. It's normal to react with sadness and concern after a diagnosis of a chronic, serious, or terminal illness, but it's abnormal to react as though your life were over.

As I described in the previous chapter, the best approach to living well is to make the most of what you have while you have it, even when it's not what you originally hoped for. This means that even though your very real and challenging health condition may impose limits on your daily living, or shorten your lifespan, you still owe it to yourself to work hard to overcome your illness anxiety so you can enjoy every good moment that you have in your life. A friend who experiences severe migraines tells me that she would rather host a birthday party for her child while having a severe migraine than not have any children or miss attending her children's birthday parties. The pain cannot take the joy of living away from her.

You might also justify your illness anxiety by believing that anyone in your shoes would be anxious and worried. This assumption is also incorrect. Research conducted by Kelly McGonigal and others (2015) shows that people who thrive under adversity actually *improve* their coping and discover deeper and more meaningful aspects of living—directly from their experience of living with adversity—which they feel are a blessing. Conversely, her research also showed that those who viewed the stressors of their lives as being bad, a punishment, or a tragedy were the ones most likely to crumble emotionally and physically.

Any patient-oriented website dedicated to a serious or terminal illness will direct people to get treatment for anxiety, because although it's an understandable response, it's a maladaptive response. If you have illness anxiety about your serious or terminal illness, it will rob you of the ability to perceive the good moments that are present in your daily life.

It's more likely that you came into your illness with the tendency to develop anxiety, as opposed to your illness causing you to become anxious. The problem is the way you view your circumstances. Although your illness or condition may be a problem and a trigger for your anxiety, it's not *the* problem. Worry about your illness is the problem. And it's a problem that is guaranteed to make you unnecessarily miserable, even in your good moments. It has the capacity to rob you of the joy and blessings that could be yours on most days, even when your health suffers.

Real Crisis Versus Imagined Crisis

Your anxiety makes your brain accidentally react to any trigger related to illness as though it's a catastrophe—whether or not it is. If you're not aware of this tendency, then it's easy to react to every aspect of your illness or condition as though it's a crisis, whether it's getting a lab test, visiting the doctor, or undergoing treatment. It's like going to a school that has a naughty child who repeatedly pulls the fire alarm so class can stop and be interrupted. If you happen to be sensitive to this false alarm, then you jump and react as though a real fire has broken out, even when there's no smoke or flames.

RAISE YOUR RESILIENCE: Illness anxiety is like having a faulty fire alarm that goes off when there's no fire. This false alarm can make you accidentally view your circumstances as tragic, because the crisis warning is repeatedly being triggered. You may end up feeling as though you're a victim in your life, rather than a powerful agent of change. But you can also work to not react to the false alarm; to not believe the feeling that something terrible is about to happen. Notice what happens when you don't react.

To help you overcome the tendency to react to any reminder of illness as though it's a catastrophe, you need to learn to distinguish between a real crisis and an imagined crisis. This may sound obvious when you're calm, but for many with illness anxiety, it's difficult to remember this when your worry gets triggered and your body feels full of anxiety.

It helps to take the same view that medical professionals take when confronted with signs of illness and injury. They have a triage system for determining which things are real emergencies that require immediate attention and which things are those that need attention but are not life-threatening. Being worried is not useful for them, when working with sick people, because it clouds their perception and decision-making abilities.

Ways to Identify a Real Crisis

Let's review the symptoms that any medical professional would agree *are* a crisis. This list covers almost any type of situation that you might encounter in your home or out in the world. If these symptoms occur to you, you should call for emergency transport and get to the emergency room as quickly as possible.

THINGS DOCTORS CONSIDER AN EMERGENCY

Doctors are very clear about what constitutes a real emergency. If any of the following things happen to you, you need to call for emergency help and seek immediate medical care.

- Absence of a heartbeat
- Absence of breathing
- Difficulty breathing with signs of lack of oxygen, such as bluish skin or nailbeds
- Bones sticking out of your skin
- Loss of consciousness that is not explained by a known condition, such as low blood pressure or a dysautonomia
- Blood squirting out
- Amputation of a part of your body
- Sudden onset of paralysis, or partial paralysis
- Extreme acute pain
- Sudden choking that results in inability to talk or breathe
- Second-degree burns of the entire hand, foot, or genitals (blisters have formed)
- Third-degree burns of any type (skin is charred and tissue has been destroyed and smells burned)
- Sudden loss of ability to speak, to move, or to understand what others are saying
- Sudden severe fatigue or weakness that makes exertion impossible or extremely difficult

- Severe weakness where moving is difficult and makes you feel exhausted or out of breath
- Prolonged vomiting/diarrhea (more than three episodes), especially when it results in severe lethargy

The aforementioned symptoms require immediate care and it will be obvious to everyone that something is terribly wrong. Other symptoms may require medical attention, or even urgent care, but they are not at the same level of concern as those listed here. These symptoms require that you or others take immediate action, and they can properly be called a crisis.

This guideline is similar to the ones that medical staff use to determine who gets seen immediately and who is asked to wait. You can download this list here: www.newharbinger.com/49043. You may want to print it out so you have a reminder of what the real crises are in your life, to stand in opposition to your anxious version of a crisis. This checklist will help remind you that, in most if not all cases, you're experiencing a false alarm.

The problem I see in most people with illness anxiety is that they get scared by the in-between symptoms and get so befuddled with worry and anxiety that they seek reassurance by calling the doctor or going to the emergency room. When medical doctors refer their patients to me, it is usually because their patients are confusing normal, non-dangerous symptoms with those of a true emergency.

You might be asking yourself, "How do I know for sure that I have a crisis symptom? What if my arm doesn't feel right and it feels like I can't move it properly?" or "What if I'm not sure I lost consciousness? How will I know for sure?" Here's the easy answer: You'll have no doubt at all about these symptoms if they happen to you. No one else will have any doubt either.

If you have any doubt, then you can be sure that your illness anxiety is fooling you and sending out a false alarm. Doubt is a signal that nothing serious is medically wrong. It's also a signal that the big thing that is wrong is your worry about illness. Your anxiety is imagining the worst-case scenario and making it seem real.

RAISE YOUR RESILIENCE: So that the list feels personal to you, feel free to add items to the list of real medical crises offered here. You might add things that most people would consider to be a crisis, such as the death of someone they love, or being involved in a severe car accident. If you have a serious health condition, be sure to add in any special circumstances related to your health condition that your medical team have told you is a crisis in need of immediate medical attention. Then, whenever your alarm bells go off, you can check this list to discover if they're real or not.

EXCEPTIONS TO THE RULE

Sometimes there are exceptions. You might be like Jimmy, who had severe allergies that easily triggered anaphylactic shock, a life-threatening reaction. He carried a special injection pen that he or others could use if he suspected accidental exposure to peanuts or eggs. His doctors wanted him to always go to the nearest emergency department anytime he suspected an exposure to peanuts or eggs, because his body had such a severe allergic reaction. This meant that he sometimes had some false alarms, but his health care team knew that it was too dangerous to risk not getting immediate emergency help. As another example, people who are prone to heart attacks are not able to increase the workload on their heart by doing some kinds of exercise, running up stairs, or even walking vigorously. People prone to strokes lose the ability to function in a certain area of the body, no matter how hard they try.

If you're still not sure whether your health is in crisis, clarify with your health care provider which situations require an emergency response, what signs they use to decide when someone requires immediate medical attention.

If you repeatedly worry that you're having a stroke and you believe that you just felt weird and weak in your left arm, but you can still hold your phone or a glass of water, then you need to remind yourself to do some exposure practice and avoid calling for an ambulance, even if you have known heart disease. You can tell yourself, "This is just a false alarm.

It's not a real crisis. This is my anxiety getting triggered. I need to slow down, stop seeking reassurance and just leave things alone."

If you think that you might have fainted, but you don't find yourself waking up on the floor or draped over nearby furniture, then you need to assume that you're okay, and your illness anxiety is trying to fool you into believing that something is wrong when everything is fine.

The rule here is to get guidance and clarity when you have a real health condition, and then to not improve upon what your health care provider told you to do. If you have been told that you are in good health, or been told by a medical professional that a symptom that made you consult them is of no consequence, then you need to assume that it is your anxiety that is the problem.

Chronic Illness

When you have a chronic or serious illness, you're faced with something that may be difficult to accept. This is now your new normal. If you get stuck in feeling victimized by your condition, or if you consider your life to be tragic, then this idea of your health condition being "normal" may seem impossible to embrace. You may think my suggestion is flippant, or one of those things that is easily said by someone who has never been in your shoes. It most definitely is not.

When I gave birth to my first son, I imagined raising a child who resembled the many people in my family who had graduate degrees and were talented at sports or the arts. I also wanted to enjoy my son and being a mother. I had enjoyed my family and upbringing and I imagined the same for myself. I also came from a long line of women who had relatively easy pregnancies and births, so it never occurred to me that my experience would be different than theirs.

My first pregnancy was a nightmare of constant and severe vomiting, severe asthma, pneumonia, and tears in my placenta that threatened the life of my unborn son. I was grateful just to survive pregnancy with both myself and my son still alive and breathing.

Unfortunately, my son was born with cerebral palsy, severe learning disabilities, and several other diagnoses. I did my best to help him get all the therapy he needed; I was determined to be a heroic mother who was up to the job of creating a fun life for our family, a mom who enjoyed her family and whose family enjoyed her. I was able to remain fairly optimistic and worry-free—until my son turned eleven.

At eleven years old, cyclic vomiting syndrome struck and brought our family's life to a halt. Cyclic vomiting is a horrible condition that is considered to be the most severe and painful of the vomiting disorders. My son projectile-vomited every two to three minutes for three months straight, until he received the correct diagnosis and treatment that began to decrease his symptoms.

As you might expect, I was grief-stricken at the news of my son having another serious condition, added to his already existing disabilities. I viewed his life as tragic and unfair. I began having daytime worries about his death and nightmares about him never recovering from cyclic vomiting. I resented all of the mothers who took for granted their child's good health and normal development. I became afraid to operate his intravenous medicine, because I worried that I would accidentally inject an air bubble that might kill him.

At some point during the dark days of cyclic vomiting, my husband put up a wall plaque that said WELCOME TO CAMP RUN AMOK. This sign perfectly expressed the everyday reality of my family and it made me laugh. When I realized the only version of my son that I would get is the one that had, in effect, run amok from my fantasy of a son, I laughed. The only version of my son that was possible was the version that included disabilities, weird symptoms, and lots of visits to medical specialists.

The New Normal

Reframing my son's struggle as being the new normal made it so much easier to ignore the urge to worry or to view his life as tragic or unfair. His life *was* normal for him and our family. We were not a constant crisis waiting to happen. We were just very familiar and experienced with all the things that people with disabilities and chronic illness experience, like a trauma surgeon is used to lots of near-death situations.

Being able to use the idea of the new normal also made it much easier to calmly accept and manage the situation when my son's younger brother later developed cyclic vomiting syndrome. It gave my son and my family a new dignity that embraced our way of being in the world, without unfairly comparing ourselves to others who were not like us. When my second child developed cyclic vomiting symptoms, I felt glad to know what to do and how to cope. This was my family's version of normal and we would not be in the world without these conditions. Therefore, why treat it as a tragedy or a crisis?

When you decide to view your health condition as the new normal, you're fighting back against the temptation to be a maximizer about your health (as I described in Chapter 5) and to unfairly compare your circumstances with an imagined ideal that is never attainable. You restore your dignity as you embrace your version of humanity in all its complications.

If you have diabetes, then wearing an insulin pump is your new normal. If you have cancer, then getting chemotherapy or radiation on a regular basis is your new normal. If you have a condition that requires frequent monitoring, then being on a first-name basis with all of the lab staff is your new normal. Whatever it is that you have to monitor, manage, and experience because of your health condition is normal for you. It's just something that you have to take into account when you go about your day. It's your version of all the things that people have to adapt to because of something outside of their control.

All of us have something that requires us to adapt and shift our perspective away from our imagined ideal of a life without suffering or challenges. If you're short, then you need a step stool to reach the top cabinets. If you have red hair and fair skin, then you have to wear sunscreen and protective clothing to avoid getting sick from sunburn.

Just as you would not feel sorry for people who are short, or who are unable to tan, you should not feel sorry for yourself when you experience a health condition that imposes restrictions on your life. Reframing your medical condition as being your new normal grants you the dignity that comes with coping with normal human limitations, instead of pushing you toward pathos and self-pity.

The beauty of living comes from learning to appreciate what you have because you adapted to life's challenges. Think about it. If you have ever raised or worked with young children, then you know the beauty of the uninterrupted quiet, still moment in which no one needs anything, cries, tantrums, or does something naughty. If everything went according to plan, you would have no perspective or appreciation for the lovely, joyful, or peaceful moments.

Even if you have a terminal illness, you'll benefit from viewing your status as the new normal of your life. You should still do exposure practice and decrease your reassurance-seeking. Ironically, I have known several people who had illness anxiety that went away when they learned they were terminally ill. They told me that they no longer had any uncertainty and therefore they didn't feel the need to worry about something they could not change.

Illness Anxiety after Becoming Terminally Ill

I have also worked with people who continued to experience illness anxiety after becoming terminally ill. If you're one of these people whose anxiety about terminal illness disrupts all peace of mind, please be reassured that the techniques described in this book can work for you. You can practice exposure to your situation, your imagined awful future, and to any fears you might have that trigger your anxiety. I have seen people like you overcome their illness anxiety, so they could live the end of their life without the added frustration of anxiety.

Your goal will be to do the same exposure practice that anyone else would do, until your anxiety level is low and you can accept and tolerate the items on your list. You may have to take more gradual steps, to accommodate reduced energy or poor concentration, but exposure will work for you.

You may still experience some anxiety and sadness about your illness and end of life, but your goal will be to experience the levels of anxiety and sadness typically experienced by people who share your condition, who don't have illness anxiety. From there you can even explore ways to find the peace and acceptance that can lead to a joyful eleventh hour.

Meditation in Reply to False Alarms

In addition to exposure practice, you can counter the physical and mental side effects of the false alarms that illness anxiety sets off by learning to meditate. Meditation teaches your body and mind to become fully grounded in the present moment, as it is, without being distracted by the "what if" or "should have" thoughts that underlie anxiety.

The benefits of learning to meditate are extensive and include calming your nervous system, releasing feel-good hormones, lowering your blood pressure, and inducing a calm, focused state—the opposite of what you feel when you're worrying about health (Goyal et al. 2014).

Meditation's greatest benefit for you is that returning your mind to the present offers you a better chance of realizing whether you have a real health problem or an imagined problem. Being able to return your mind to the present also helps you notice what is good in the present, instead of always being distracted by illness anxiety's imagined awful future.

If you have a health condition you must manage, being able to focus upon the present moment makes it easier to accept your condition as part of your new normal, because you take yourself out of catastrophe mode. Research shows that learning to meditate works well to decrease anxiety and worry. It's worth taking the time to learn.

There are so many wonderful methods for meditating, you're guaranteed to find one that suits your personal needs. I have never been able to sit in lotus pose, not even as a young child, but I adore walking or moving in nature while mindfully focusing upon my surroundings or my breathing. It's also easier for me to meditate when I listen to a guided meditation, where someone leads me through it. Conversely, I really dislike trying to sit alone and meditate quietly on my own. The trick is finding what works for you.

Another key to meditation is learning not to evaluate, or judge, what happens while you're meditating. All practice is good practice, no matter how much your mind wanders or how poorly you think you did. The end goal is to learn to suspend all judgment of yourself, the situation, and your experience while you completely focus on your inner experience. One way to do this is through open-minded curiosity. There are many excellent resources to help you learn to meditate, and I list some in the Resources section at the back of this book.

Following are some simple ways that you can practice meditating. Make it a goal to do this for five to ten minutes a day at the start, and then increase by five minutes each week until you build up to twenty minutes a day. You can also use peaceful music (perhaps the sound of the ocean surf or the wind in the pines), a meditation app like Insight Timer, or no background sound at all. Be willing to experiment with what allows you to bring your awareness into a nonjudgmental, nonanalytical focus on the experience. Meditation is great practice for simply being fully aware in the present. This feeling of being fully aware also helps you to feel fully alive and open to the experience of the present, regardless of the state of your health. What a wonderful opportunity!

EXERCISE Sitting or Lying Down Meditation

Set a timer for the amount of time you wish to practice, so you don't have to pay attention to the time. Get into a comfortable position, either sitting or lying down. Keep your legs and arms uncrossed and unclenched, with palms extended open and outward. If you're familiar with yoga, lay in corpse pose, also called shavasana: lying flat with your legs and arms straight open at your sides, with both your arms and legs rotating slightly outward.

Close your eyes and bring your attention to your breathing, breathing in and out through your mouth as quietly and gently as possible. Try to keep your attention solely focused upon your breath, the sensations of your belly rising and falling and the feel of the air gently going in and out of your lungs.

When your mind gets distracted by thoughts, plans, or worries, gently bring your attention back to your breathing. Don't worry about how often your mind wanders from your breathing. Wandering is normal—the important thing is, when you notice you've wandered away, to gently bring yourself back.

EXERCISE Favorite Place Meditation

Make yourself comfortable. Imagine visiting your favorite place. Picture the sights, one by one. Smell the air. Notice how your skin, hair, and body feel. Walk or move around in your favorite place and take the time to savor each new thing or person you see. When your mind wanders, gently bring it back to your favorite place.

Notice every detail, one by one—how it feels, looks, smells; the colors, textures, surroundings. Take your time examining everything that you see in this place. Be like an anthropologist seeing a new place and a new culture for the first time and notice every detail. Notice your body's reaction to being there. What happens to your muscles, your breath, your emotions, your posture? Take your time fully experiencing and enjoying being in this special place.

EXERCISE Moving Meditation

Find a path, trail, or, if you have access to one, a labyrinth. Set your timer for your intended practice time. Gently walk on the path while focusing all of your attention on the sensation of your body walking, the feel of the path beneath your feet, the air around you, the sounds and smells.

Walk at a pace that feels comfortable and easy. This is not an exercise session. It's a time to mindfully pay attention to what it's like to be moving through your environment without judgment, hurry, or purpose, other than to fully immerse yourself in the experience of being there. When your mind wanders, bring it back to the sensation of walking, or to the feel of the sun on your skin, the air moving across your skin, or the sights around you.

Notice how your muscles feel. Notice your breathing. Notice your reaction to moving and the feel of the path beneath your feet. Do this until your practice time is finished. Again, use a timer or plan to walk a certain distance so you don't have to keep track of the time.

There are many free apps and recordings of various meditations that you can use to keep things interesting or find a new method. An online search will show you many options and it should be easy to find something that works well for you. Take the time to find a style of meditation that suits you.

Managing Real Risks

If you happen to have a chronic or serious health condition, you might find it difficult to develop helpful ways to protect your health without crossing over the line into reassurance-seeking. For example, during the COVID-19 pandemic you might have been told by your doctor to quarantine and observe strict social distancing because of a chronic or serious health condition. You might have found it difficult to go outside your home, get groceries, or to handle delivered packages because you feared contracting COVID-19.

If you get into a chronically anxious state about avoiding exposure to any transmittable virus or disease, and feel as though all contact with anything outside your home is like going into a toxic wasteland, then your illness anxiety may be hijacking your good intentions and your health care provider's instructions. The problem is figuring out what is medically necessary in order to feel certain that you have avoided all risk of contamination.

Robert's Story

Robert was referred to me after his wife insisted that he talk to a therapist. Robert has an autoimmune condition that requires taking medicine that suppresses his immune system. This places him at high risk for complications if he contracts any viral illness, especially COVID-19.

When Robert had to leave the house during the pandemic, he used two face masks instead of one, a face shield, and his eyeglasses. He wore double pairs of gloves, in case the top layer got punctured, and carried a large bottle of hand sanitizer that he used copiously to clean his gloved hands every time he had to touch a surface. He also avoided standing within eight to ten feet of any other people, to avoid contact with any virus droplets.

When he returned home, he had to leave all his clothing in the garage before he entered the house to take a shower, using the kind of soap surgeons use to cleanse skin before operating. He also would not allow anyone to open any groceries or other delivered items for three days, until he believed no possible virus could survive. Robert told me that his doctor approved of his extreme measures. So, what could possibly be wrong with this scenario?

The problem is that anxiety ended up setting the standard for avoidance and cleaning instead of reasonable science. Discussion with Robert's doctor revealed that his doctor thought Robert was actually overdoing it with safety measures, but since no one could be sure what the safest things were to do, he was willing to agree with Robert's protocol—though he certainly didn't tell his other patients to double up with personal protective equipment or to shower with expensive surgical soap. His specialty was the endocrine system, and he didn't realize the high cost that avoidance and reassurance-seeking had inflicted on Robert's mental health.

Robert had been choosing to live by unnecessarily rigid and extreme rules that were beyond the recommendations of his doctor, and had found other YouTube videos of doctors recommending extreme procedures, which he used as proof that he should do the same. Robert tried to eliminate all risk by taking extreme measures.

No matter what medical condition you might have, you need to learn to gracefully accept that you cannot eliminate all risks. It's good enough to follow your health care team's guidelines, without embellishment. You can be content with their recommendations and do not need to improve upon them by doing additional research and finding more conservative guidelines to follow.

Here are a few helpful tips to help you to follow your doctor's instructions, while avoiding anxiety-promoting behaviors.

1. Don't research the validity of your health care team's special guidelines for your medical condition. Assume that the information they give you is useful and valid.

2. Accept that you'll need to take risks in order to live a mentally and physically well life. If you're afraid of going outside due to a pandemic or even seasonal flu outbreaks, wear a mask and any other protective equipment your doctor suggests and go for a walk, to the grocery store, or the park. Enjoy what you can and don't subtract things from your life unless your doctor tells you to. Aim to live well instead of to avoid all risks.

3. Remember that your mental health is part of your overall health. You need to attend to your mental health as much as your physical health. People who socialize, exercise, spend time outdoors, get sunlight, and have daily ways to be productive and enjoy hobbies are the healthiest. Anxiety that is out of control is never good for your mental or physical health.

Having a chronic or serious medical condition doesn't have to be a barrier to overcoming your illness anxiety. You can learn to distinguish between the false alarm of illness anxiety and the real need to attend to your health. Having a condition doesn't disqualify you from mastering your anxiety. It may require some adaptations to take an attitude that views your life as beautiful, meaningful, and heroic, in which you choose to rise to the occasion of living well by mastering your anxiety.

Please don't allow your illness anxiety to place further limitations on your life, *especially* if you suffer from a serious health condition. If you have a serious or chronic health condition, that alone is a reminder that life is precious and sometimes fragile. Therefore, it's incumbent upon you to do all that you can to enjoy it and live as fully as possible. That means embracing uncertainty and risk with great gusto as you do your exposure practice.

CHAPTER 7

Enhancing Your Recovery

Have you ever had one of those days where everything you do to push back your illness anxiety seems to fail? Do you ever feel like you're making progress, and feel pleased that news about other people's health problems no longer triggers your anxiety, only to crumble when you notice a random physical sensation, such as feeling unexpectedly hot and sweaty? If so, then you might be struggling like Aubrey.

Aubrey's Story

Aubrey's doctor wanted me to help her (and him) because she called him almost every week worrying about fevers and chills. Aubrey told me that she was constantly worrying that she and her children had unexplained fevers that might be a symptom of leukemia. She had known a family in her community who lost both a young child and an uncle to an unusually virulent form of leukemia, and dreaded that this might happen to herself and her children.

Aubrey had learned that the two people who had died had experienced nighttime sweats and fevers. This alarmed her because she had noticed that when she nursed her children at night, or checked on them, sometimes they were hot and sweaty, and the same went for herself. She also worried that she was getting overheated and sweating too much at exercise class, or when walking rapidly, and noticed random episodes of perspiration.

She started carrying a thermometer and checking her temperature whenever she felt warm or perspired, and she noticed that sometimes her temperature was higher than the average normal temperature. She did the same temperature tracking for her children, to the point that her older children protested whenever they saw her approaching with a thermometer, or leaning in to touch their foreheads with the back of her hand. She frequently called the doctor to verify that any thermometer readings higher than 98.6°F/37.2°C were safe and not indicative of leukemia —even though her doctor and her children's pediatrician had told her to stop calling for any fevers below 103°F/39.4°C.

Things really got difficult for Aubrey when she began to avoid exercising, walking up the stairs, walking briskly, or letting her children get overheated. She recalled her grandmother warning her to "not let the children get all sweated up because it might make them sick." This seemed to add credence to her fear that an elevated body temperature was a dangerous symptom.

Aubrey began getting panic attacks when she felt warm, perspired, or whenever she didn't feel perfectly well and full of energy. She began avoiding taking her own pulse or blood pressure, because doing this caused a panic attack. Furthermore, the more she lost fitness because she avoided exercise, the more easily she got hot and sweaty doing normal daily tasks because she was out of shape. Additionally, anxiety can cause hot flashes, cold chills, increased heart rate, and benign increases in blood pressure, the very sensations that she feared.

Aubrey's problem was not just worrying about illness, it was also about reacting to the physical sensations of normal living and anxiety. She was scared of feeling scared and scared of noticing any changes in her body, even when they were perfectly normal.

Doug's Story

Or you might identify with Doug, who worried about getting a serious bowel disorder, such as celiac, ulcerative colitis, or cancer. Every time he felt his stomach rumble or noticed some cramping or bloating, he became anxious and worried that he was developing a chronic and serious bowel condition. If he felt full after a meal or snack, he got panicky that he would never be able to eat comfortably again.

Doug began eating bland foods, the kind recommended after a bout of vomiting, in order to avoid creating gut sensations such as nausea, gas, and signs of digestion. He only ate food in small quantities and lost a lot of weight, even though he was really hungry and wanted to eat more food. He avoided fizzy drinks, because they made him burp and pass gas, which triggered worry and panic attacks. Even though he had been tested for signs of bowel disease and had been told by his doctor that his gut was "very healthy," he lived in daily fright that something was seriously wrong each time he noticed any gut sensations.

Unfortunately for Doug, anxiety often creates lots of gut sensations that can include GI pain, cramping, diarrhea, nausea, bloating, and rumbling. Just like Aubrey, he was in a bind: his anxiety was creating the very symptoms that he dreaded. They both suffered from high levels of anxiety sensitivity, the fear of feeling afraid.

If you can identify with Aubrey or Doug and you dread the physical sensations of your body because they make you fear that you're seriously ill, then please pay close attention to the information in this chapter. I'll introduce you to a powerful tool to boost the effectiveness of your exposure practice: interoceptive exposure.

Re-Create the Sensations You Fear Most

Interoceptive exposure is a type of exposure practice that focuses on re-creating the physical sensations that trigger your anxiety and worry (Busscher et al. 2012, Sabourin et al. 2015). Instead of re-creating a situation that provokes anxiety, such as reading medical information or having your blood pressure taken, interoceptive exposure re-creates the sensations that provoke fear.

In Chapters 4, 5, and 6, you practiced facing situations and thoughts that you avoid or endure with dread. In this chapter, you'll learn how to face the physical sensations that trigger your worry and increase your anxiety about illness. It's a way to be more precise in targeting all of the things that play into your anxiety about illness.

RAISE YOUR RESILIENCE: Being willing to do interoceptive exposure in combination with your other exposure practice powers up the intensity of your practice. For example, if you fear dying from a heart attack, running up several flights of stairs to raise your heart rate while imagining you're having a heart attack helps you to learn to ignore the false alarm signals from both your mind and your body. Combining techniques helps you master your illness anxiety faster.

Do I Have Anxiety Sensitivity?

If you have anxiety sensitivity, then you'll feel afraid of what happens to your body and your mind when you get anxious (Zvolensky et al. 2018). You'll react strongly to changes in sensation when you're anxious, and may mistake these sensations for a sign that something is seriously wrong. You'll also tend to believe that it's both physically and mentally dangerous to be anxious. You might also have the misconception that really healthy people never feel the physical symptoms of anxiety, and that calm and healthy people always feel great.

Here are some examples of the types of things that you might think if you have high anxiety sensitivity:

- *It scares me when I feel anxious*
- *It scares me when I feel my heartbeat, especially if it gets faster or stronger*
- *It scares me if I get out of breath*
- *It scares me if I feel lightheaded or dizzy*
- *It scares me if I feel shaky*
- *It scares me if I perspire or feel hot*

In contrast, people who are low on anxiety sensitivity dislike feeling anxious or feeling sick, but they don't get alarmed about feeling that way. They tend to take a practical approach to noticing the sensations of their body. They might notice that they feel anxious, but instead of getting alarmed, their inner dialogue goes something like this, *Hmm...I must be a bit stressed, because my stomach is so upset and I can tell that my heart is beating faster.* Then they turn their attention to the next thing at hand and forget about what they felt in their body. They don't feel distracted by the sensations of their body and they view them as neutral events to be endured, but not scrutinized or checked. They have a "How about that?" attitude that is both accepting of the sensation and validating of their emotion, and then they move on to the next important thing that really matters to their long-term goal of living a good life.

This may seem hard to imagine, but you too can get to the same point that people low in anxiety sensitivity experience.

RAISE YOUR RESILIENCE: Interoceptive exposure can teach you to take an accepting and nonjudgmental attitude toward physical sensations. Try to become open-minded and curious about what you feel, instead of getting stuck on the worst-case scenario.

The Science of How Treatment Works

Scientists have discovered that if you have anxiety sensitivity, you risk incomplete recovery if you do not treat it directly (Oser et al. 2019, Sabourin et al. 2015). You must add interoceptive exposure into your treatment in order to guarantee a full recovery. As explained in Chapter 3, anxiety sensitivity is the fear of feeling the physical sensations of anxiety. This means you have an extra problem to tackle: learning to accept and get comfortable with all the sensations that happen to a human body when the anxiety response gets triggered.

Your body has an oversensitive alarm system for noticing internal bodily changes. You're also at a much higher risk for getting an anxious reaction to any internal change, even when it's not directly related to anxiety (McLeish et al. 2015, Avallone and McLeish 2014, Zvolenshy et al. 2001). The rub is that your anxiety will cause physical sensations, many of which can easily be confused with symptoms of illness. Anxiety has the capacity to create a vast array of sensations that you might not easily recognize as being due to anxiety. Here is a list of benign anxiety sensations that can happen one at a time or in random clusters:

- GI sensations: nausea, vomiting, gagging, dry heaving, diarrhea, feeling the sudden need to defecate, cramping, rumbling, butterflies feeling
- Heart sensations: sudden increase in heartbeats, elevated heartbeats while at rest, sudden sensation of a very loud or skipped heartbeat
- Breathing sensations: not being able to catch your breath while at rest, a feeling of needing more air, tight chest
- Hot flashes, cold chills, and sweating
- Feeling shaky; hands, arms, and legs feeling shaky
- Numbness in your hands, arms, feet, and legs, or even in your face (*parathesias*)
- Feeling dizzy, lightheaded, or like you might faint
- Things seeming surreal; feeling out-of-body or out-of-place
- Inner sensation of trembling, an electric feeling inside
- Feeling as though you're dying or going insane
- Fatigue and feeling weak, like it's difficult to move or think
- Headaches, shooting pains in your arms or legs, due to chronically tight muscles that impinge your nerve fibers

You might have confused some of these symptoms with those of a serious disorder and then gotten stuck in a downward spiral of checking for symptoms, noticing symptoms, seeking reassurance, getting more anxious, and then doing it all over again. How frustrating!

Additionally, you might be doing things to avoid creating physical symptoms because you feel terrified when you notice a certain pain, a certain feeling, or something that seems not quite right. Your problem might not be fearing anxiety symptoms in general; it may be centered around fear of anything specific to the illness you fear.

When others feel afraid, they can handle feeling anxious without worrying about it—for example, athletes who know they always get nervous before a game, but don't worry about it or find it to be a problem. In your case, you'll also need to do interoceptive exposure, to stop getting triggered by feared sensations you equate with serious illness. Here is a list of typical examples of this type of fear:

- Being afraid of noticing your heartbeats because it makes you think about heart attacks
- Being afraid to eat high fiber because it makes you feel full, bloated, and rumbly, and this in turn reminds you of cancer or GI illnesses
- Being afraid of headaches because they remind you of brain tumors
- Being afraid of perspiration at night because it reminds you of blood cancers
- Being afraid of fatigue because it reminds you of cancer or wasting diseases
- Being afraid of trembling because it reminds you of Parkinson's disease
- Being afraid of getting overheated, cold, or exercising too much, because it reminds you of getting sick
- Being afraid of getting lightheaded, dizzy, or feeling not quite yourself because it reminds you of going insane

- Being afraid of losing your concentration or not remembering something because it reminds you of dementia
- Being afraid to rub your hand over your body, for fear you'll find a tumor

As you can see from both of these lists, we'll need to direct your attention toward losing your fear of these sensations and disconnecting the automatic worry and anxiety response that occurs when you notice them.

This is why interoceptive exposure can power up your recovery. It gives you a way to directly address all the sensations you fear, and to teach your body how to stand down from its automatic anxious response when it notices an internal change. Scientists have discovered that practicing interoceptive exposure will improve your treatment when you have anxiety sensitivity (Busscher et al. 2012).

How to Make Interoceptive Practice Work for You

First, you need to use the same procedures for practicing interoceptive exposure that you use for practicing any other type of exposure. You can use the same worksheets (available here: www.newharbinger.com/49043) you have been using in the previous chapters, only this time your exposure practice will focus on creating the physical sensations that provoke your anxiety. You'll want to notice the thoughts and level of anxiety you experience prior to your interoceptive exposure, and then after your practice (the learned inhibition technique). Let me describe how interoceptive exposure practice looked for Jessica, who was afraid of having a heart attack or a stroke.

Jessica's Story

Jessica is middle-aged and has always been told by her doctor that she is in good health. But her anxiety makes her afraid of noticing her heartbeats, feeling out of breath, and of overexerting herself, in case her heart is not as strong as it should be.

She warms up very slowly when she exercises and slows down or rests if she gets out of breath or cannot talk while exercising. She also dislikes taking her pulse, because she is afraid that it will be too high and therefore make her even more anxious. She also avoids starting any physical activity rapidly for fear of having a heart attack or stroke. She dreads getting her blood pressure taken, because it's always a bit too high and she has been told that she has "white coat hypertension"—which occurs only when the doctor or nurse takes her blood pressure, but otherwise her blood pressure is assumed to be normal.

For her interoceptive exposure practice, Jessica chose running in place, going up a flight of stairs rapidly, and doing jumping jacks as methods for inducing a rapid heartbeat, feeling out of breath, and feeling like she might induce a heart attack or a stroke. She also agreed to do these exposure practices without engaging in a slow, careful warm-up beforehand.

Before Jessica began her interoceptive practice, she wrote of her level of anticipatory anxiety: "This feels so dangerous. I don't know if I can do it. What if I really do have a heart attack or a stroke? What made me agree to do this dangerous activity?" Then she did five jumping jacks without warming up. She felt really scared and then did ten more jumping jacks, after I encouraged her to keep going. She told me, "I cannot believe that I'm doing this! I have not done fifteen jumping jacks in years!" Then after a minute of rest, before she could catch her breath, she did twenty-five more jumping jacks. She reported that she was more out of breath than she could recall in the many years she had been scared of exercising —she felt both scared and excited by this.

Next, I had her go to the stairwell and quickly run up a flight of stairs as fast as she could, without catching her breath from the jumping jacks. We repeated this ten times in a row, each time with me asking her if she thought she could do another flight, and whether or not she was feeling just out of breath and out of shape, or if she really was having symptoms of a heart attack or stroke.

I also asked her to pay attention to how vigorously and rapidly her heart was beating, instead of avoiding awareness of her heartbeats. I even asked her to see if she could get her heart rate to beat out of control (which she could not).

After this, she realized that nothing terrible was happening. She realized she was managing her anxiety and doing vigorous exercise without a warm-up and was still just fine. Then she ran in place, to see if she could actually cause a panic attack, heart attack, or stroke. She ran until she could not talk or sing, and then for two more minutes, to test her fear that vigorous exercise would actually be deadly or unbearable. She ran in place while taking her neck pulse, to help her pay close attention to the feeling of rapid heartbeats. Whenever her heartbeats got slower, she did more running in place to make them faster.

The interoceptive exposure practice ended when Jessica realized that vigorous exercise and noticing her heartbeats was way less scary that she initially thought it would be. She learned that the worst thing that happened was feeling out of breath—not having a heart attack, panic attack, or stroke.

Jessica also learned that her anticipatory anxiety was inaccurate and not worth listening to the next time, because it predicted the exact opposite of what happened during her practice. She had predicted that she would not be able to do vigorous exercise and that she surely would experience a terrible panic attack. She also incorrectly predicted that her fear would increase the more she exercised. She was surprised to discover that the more she exercised and paid attention to her heartbeats, the less frightened she felt.

Jessica learned that her fear of heart attack and stroke decreased, along with her fear of noticing cardiac sensations—simply by daring to induce the sensations she feared and paying close attention to these sensations until she lost her fear.

How Do I Create Different Sensations for Interoceptive Exposure?

Figuring out how to create the sensations you fear might be obvious in some situations, such as Jessica's, where simply exercising and checking your pulse is the best approach. Other situations, such as feeling feverish, might not be so easy to figure out. Let me give you some ideas that therapists use when they are helping their clients do interoceptive exposure.

If you fear rapid heartbeats, try this:

- Running in place, jumping jacks, walking up and down stairs
- Taking your pulse
- Listening to your heartbeats with a stethoscope (these can be purchased from a local pharmacy or online)

If you fear being out of breath, try this:

- Breathing through a straw, a snorkel with mask, a coffee stirrer
- Running in place, jumping jacks, walking up and down stairs
- Breathing underwater through a snorkel, in your tub or in a hot tub or pool

If you fear feeling hot and feverish, try this:

- Wearing several heavy sweaters or sweatshirts and sweatpants
- Turning up the heat in your house and doing exercise or chores that require lots of movement, such as vacuuming
- Eating hot peppers
- Sitting in your car with the heat turned up too high
- Vigorous exercise in the sun or on a hot day
- Sitting in a sauna
- Taking a long hot shower and then putting on too-warm clothes

If you fear feeling jittery, try this:

- Drinking two cups of regular coffee
- Drinking several caffeinated soft drinks

If you fear feeling dizzy or lightheaded, try this:

- Spinning in a desk chair
- Spinning on your own (with a spotter, so you don't fall)
- Hyperventilating: breathing in and out rapidly until you feel dizzy and woozy

If you fear sensations in your belly or gut, try this:

- Eat too much food and then drink a fizzy beverage and jump up and down
- Eat a high-fiber meal with lots of beans and gas-producing veggies, such as broccoli and cauliflower
- Drink caffeinated beverages to induce gut activity, called peristalsis
- Take a laxative if you fear diarrhea, but only for the purpose of doing exposure practice
- Eat foods that you're afraid to eat, unless you get an anaphylactic or severe allergic response

If you fear you might go insane, or not feel in control of your mind, try this:

- Hyperventilating: breathing in and out rapidly until you feel dizzy and woozy
- Hyperventilating until you feel woozy and then trying to solve difficult math problems, crosswords, or Sudoku puzzles

If you're afraid of getting cold, try this:

- Going barefoot during cool weather
- Not wearing warm-enough clothes during cool weather
- Placing ice packs on your feet, hands, armpits, and the back of your neck until you feel chilled
- Soaking in a cold shower or bath water that is not comfortably warm
- Standing in front of an open freezer in shorts, bare feet, and a t-shirt

If you're afraid of looking sickly, try this:

- Wearing white or very pale makeup, or costume makeup, on your face (you can go online to get makeup advice about creating a ghostly or sickly pallor)
- Wearing colors that make your face and skin look pale or gray, wearing black lipstick and nail gloss

Once you can do interoceptive exposures, then you can further enhance your exposure practice by combining your interoceptive exposures with the previous types of exposure. For example, you could practice not getting reassurance while saying the thoughts you most fear *and* while hyperventilating—to try and do as much as possible to provoke your anxiety.

Using interoceptive exposure in this way is very powerful. It creates an opportunity for practice that simulates what happens when you spontaneously feel anxious about illness. In my experience, when someone is willing to combine each type of exposure into a combined exposure practice, they get the best results. Research on inhibitory learning, mentioned earlier in Chapter 3, proves this to be true (Tolin 2019).

RAISE YOUR RESILIENCE: In your journal, write down any bodily sensations that you realize trigger your anxiety about illness. If your anxiety is about someone else, make a similar list of the bodily symptoms that you fear, such as noticing someone looks pale, is perspiring, or has a heartbeat that seems too rapid. Then select a method for inducing these symptoms in either yourself, or the person whose health you worry about, and put this on your exposure practice list. Follow the previous guidelines for exposure practice, including increasing the intensity of your practice.

Creating Your Practice List

Your practice list might look something like this:

Fear of feeling feverish	1. Wear too many layers of clothes while doing housework 2. Rub muscle balm on my chest, back, and legs 3. Drink hot beverages while wearing too many clothes and using muscle balm
Fear of my children getting a fever	1. Have my kids wear "ghost" makeup after school and after baths 2. Let them run around before bedtime until they get hot and sweaty 3. Give them hot cocoa after they run around
Fear of headaches because it might be a brain tumor	1. Don't take pain meds for mild headaches 2. Eat really cold ice cream or drink a milkshake quickly so I get an "ice cream headache" 3. Coughing really hard until my head hurts

RAISE YOUR RESILIENCE: The more you're willing to expose yourself to anything you fear—including sensations, situations, and scary thoughts—the faster and more fully you'll recover.

You should now have a thorough list of all the things that you need to practice in order to overcome your illness anxiety. As you can see, there are quite a few facets to how you experience your anxiety, and they require your willingness to face them without the quick escape of reassurance-seeking, or avoiding the situation altogether. This will take courage—which is, again, defined as your ability to do the things that scare you—in order to successfully master your anxiety.

The previous seven chapters have focused on mastering and overcoming anxiety. What happens, though, when your doctor, health clinic, or the health care system play into your illness anxiety? The next chapter will help you to determine whether your health care system is accidentally promoting your anxiety.

CHAPTER 8

What to Do When Your Health Care System Accidentally Promotes Anxiety

It's true that your health care team may make it harder for you to overcome your anxiety about illness and dying. Doctors and nurses are part of a system that is built around intolerance of uncertainty, avoidance of lawsuits, and generating profit from lab tests and expensive diagnostic procedures. What does this mean for you when you get anxious about your health? Let's take a closer look.

Ordinarily we trust our health care providers to do their very best to treat our illnesses and protect us from preventable illnesses. Typically, people are drawn to the field of medicine because they love caring for people and they enjoy science and the academic study of things related to health. They must meet strict requirements for training, continuing education, and licensing that demand a high level of knowledge and high professional moral standards that put the patient first. They work hard to do their best to prevent illness and save lives, and most take great pleasure in your good health.

What happens, however, when your health care provider happens to have their own intolerance of uncertainty, or works for a health care system that fears being sued, or that rewards ordering more tests and procedures because they generate profit? Also, what happens if your health care provider believes that giving you reassurance is the best way to treat your anxiety? Each of these situations can pose an accidental roadblock in your journey to good mental and physical health.

When Your Doctor Gets Anxiety About Your Health

Health care providers can have anxiety about their patients having a serious or terminal illness, just like you have anxiety about getting seriously ill or dying. Health care professionals can have anxiety that makes them fall victim to the same pressures of negative reinforcement, reassurance-seeking, and avoidance that beset you. The difficult part is that once your doctor or nurse is out of training, they usually don't have someone looking over their shoulder to give them guidance or reassurance about making sure that you're in good health. This can create a problem for a health care provider who feels extra anxiety about getting it right and not doing any harm to their patients. They are on their own and they are just as worried as you are that nothing bad happens when you're under their care.

If your doctor or nurse is an anxiety-prone person who has excessive worry about your well-being, they can order extra tests that their non-anxious peers would not consider necessary. Your health care team has lots of negative reinforcers that are readily available to reassure both themselves and you: lab tests, diagnostic procedures, exploratory procedures, and referrals to specialists. If your doctor or nurse is seeking reassurance about your health by over-ordering labs and tests and referring you to specialists, it can become a problem for you. You might initially consider these extra tests and labs to be the mark of a thorough professional, but in the long run, you'll risk increasing your anxiety about illness.

If your doctor orders a test just to make sure, it accidentally sends the message that they are concerned about something more serious. Your anxious mind then has more reason to consider the worst-case scenario, because if the doctor really thought all was well then why order the test? Then, like most people with illness anxiety, you weaken your ability to believe in the idea that all is well, while you wait for the test results to return. Thinking about the possibility of bad news, in turn, makes you think about the worst-case scenario. Thinking about the worst-case scenario heightens your anxiety, which makes the worst-case scenario seem real and even inevitable.

Another problem with getting unnecessary tests is that no two human bodies are exactly alike. Many healthy normal people have benign tumors, slightly unusual lab results, or less common configurations in their anatomy, without suffering any ill effect. For example, when my youngest had an MRI of his skull after a bad fall, I learned that he has a common benign tumor on his pituitary gland. Had I been prone to illness anxiety and/or not already learned in graduate school that many X-rays and body scans turn up benign but unusual findings, I would have been very worried.

Additionally, when your doctor is using the idea of the average range of lab findings as a reference point, they know that the average range for a particular health condition or lab result is derived by adding together a large number of people's information and then dividing it by the number of people. That means that some of those perfectly normal and healthy people will have information that is much higher or much lower than the average. Their high or low information is not abnormal for them. It's just different from the average. This means that your doctor will be looking at a number of things, besides just a single lab or test result, to decide whether or not your test result is significant.

Many of the people I see with illness anxiety get triggered when the doctor or nurse informs them, "Your ______ reading is a little high/low, but we are just going to keep an eye on it." This is medical speak for "You're doing great, just keep getting your regular health screenings." But recently, scientists have begun to realize that individual differences are perhaps more important than averages when it comes to your health care. So you should not be alarmed when your lab or test results are a bit higher or lower than "normal."

Lucas's Story

Your doctor can get caught up in reassurance-seeking by using unnecessary lab tests. Lucas experienced this dilemma when his doctor kept ordering tests to make sure that everything was okay. Lucas liked his doctor and told me, "My doctor is really thorough and kind. He will call me at home to give me my lab results, so I don't have to wait to find out. He will go the extra mile to make sure I'm okay."

His doctor would tell him, "I just want to make sure that everything is okay. You can never be too safe." The doctor would then order extra blood tests and other procedures to rule out cancers and other dreaded diseases.

Lucas would fret with worry and lose sleep every time he got a call from his doctor's office to redo a test or get another test, to rule out things like multiple sclerosis, brain tumors, and cancer. He would get so anxious that he felt like crying and would imagine having to go into hospice each time he went to the hospital for a blood draw or other test.

His husband would repeatedly tell Lucas that Lucas was in great health and remind him that even though some of his tests were slightly off from normal, he never actually got a bad result. On some occasions, Lucas's doctor ordered repeated blood tests to verify that he was okay, because some of his results were slightly abnormal, even though they were not in the range of medical concern. These repeated tests triggered severe worry and panic attacks in Lucas, causing him to verify that his will was in order and that his husband understood his last wishes. Every visit to his doctor's office ended up being a minefield of anxiety and repeat tests.

If your doctor orders tests even though they believe everything is okay, be willing to say "No" and explain that getting an unnecessary test can make your illness anxiety worse. Ask them to only order tests when they truly believe that something is wrong, or when it's something that all doctors would order for necessary screening—based on your health risk factors, for example getting a colonoscopy once you turn fifty.

Additionally, please explain to your doctor that you have anxiety about getting illness and are learning to overcome your anxiety by not validating your worrisome thoughts that something is wrong. Explain that when your doctor orders tests just to make sure that you're okay, it creates extra challenges for you. Explain how, since your intolerance of uncertainty makes you want to constantly get proof that nothing is wrong, ordering unnecessary tests is a form of negative reinforcement that worsens your anxiety. You can tell your doctor that, therefore, you would like him or her to only order tests that are absolutely necessary.

You might also share the first three chapters and this chapter of this book with your doctor or nurse, to help them understand their patients who have anxiety about illness. If your doctor or nurse doesn't seem open to this idea, then you might want to consider finding a doctor or nurse who is interested in understanding the ways your anxiety can affect how you interact with the health care system. Most health care providers will be very interested in doing anything they can to improve your mental and physical health, if only you alert them to your concern.

Finally, if you're receiving therapy for your anxiety about illness, you can give permission for your therapist to talk with your health care provider and explain the best ways to support you in overcoming your illness anxiety. Sometimes hearing from another professional about the role of negative reinforcement and exposure practice is all your doctor needs to adjust their style of interaction. I have had this conversation many times with the health care providers of my patients and in every instance the doctor or nurse was pleased to learn how to better help the patient. They also all had correctly perceived that our mutual patient was anxious about illness and were trying their best to be helpful. They just didn't know how to be helpful and were grateful for the guidance and opportunity to coordinate care.

Academic Language Versus Layperson's Language

Do you ever have difficulty figuring out exactly what your doctor means when they talk to you? I remember listening to the pediatrician tell me "You might want to consider getting a varicella vaccination for your son.

Recent randomized controlled trials and Phase III open clinical trials of the varicella vaccine in Japanese schoolchildren show that this vaccine is efficacious approximately 85 percent of the time. The United States has not conducted any clinical trials and the American Academy of Pediatrics has yet to approve its use, but we like to offer it to our patients. What would you like to do?" Had I not spent six years in a graduate school that was part of a medical university, I would have been absolutely befuddled at their use of scientific professional language, also known as *jargon*.

My son's pediatrician was trying to be accurate and professional when speaking with me, but had I been anxious, I might have gotten confused and alarmed. I might have wondered if varicella was a serious disease, instead of understanding that it's the name for chickenpox. I might have wondered what happened to the 15 percent in whom the vaccine didn't work. Did they die? Get really sick? I could have been alarmed that the American Academy of Pediatrics had yet to endorse the vaccine for chickenpox, and started worrying about whether the vaccine was potentially dangerous. Do you see how the jargon your doctor uses can accidentally trigger your worry?

But your doctor has spent twelve to sixteen years studying scientific words and language. They worked very hard to learn and understand the specific terms that are part of scientific and medical jargon so they could be precise when communicating with other professionals. This is very important, because it prevents mistakes in research and health care, which in turn protects your health. The more quickly a health care professional masters the use of jargon, the more precise and effective they will be when working as part of a health care team.

The problem occurs when someone accidentally uses jargon with someone who is not fluent in the same jargon. It's like when I watch football with my husband, and he groans after the referee makes a call and I have to ask him to interpret the referee's call and hand signals. Since your doctor will be using jargon with his staff and colleagues for the duration of their professional life, it can be difficult to switch back and forth from jargon to everyday English.

Science relies upon the use of probability statistics. This means that any time a scientist studies a disease or treatment, they are always comparing what they are studying against what happens randomly by chance. In science, something is considered useful or important when it has a more than random chance of occurring. Medical training teaches health care professionals to think like statisticians, acknowledging that no treatment or disease has a guaranteed outcome because there's always some degree of random chance at play. This means that your doctor might feel obligated to explain what those chances are, even though the treatment is considered to be a good one.

In layperson's terms, many treatments we receive are better than not doing anything, but there's never a 100 percent guarantee. We just don't usually think or talk about that, unless we have studied science and medicine.

But if you dislike uncertainty, hearing about the percentage of people who don't respond can feel very anxiety-producing. This means that you should be assertive and explain to your health care providers that you need them to explain their diagnosis and recommendations in easy-to-understand wording, so you get a clear message. Think what it would have felt like for me to hear my pediatrician say, "There's a new chickenpox vaccine that I recommend. They have been using it in Japan for the past seven years and it's doing a great job of preventing chickenpox. You might not think chickenpox is a big deal, but it's very dangerous for adults who don't develop immunity in childhood, and it has a high risk of causing shingles in adults who had chickenpox as kids. You could spare your son the agony of shingles and help protect vulnerable adults by giving him this vaccine."

Shana's Story

Shana is an example of what can go wrong when a well-intentioned doctor gets caught up in using jargon and wanting to be clear. Shana's illness anxiety worsened after she got pregnant. She had been taking medication for her anxiety prior to getting pregnant, which her doctor recommended she continue to take, to prevent her anxiety from getting even worse.

She worried that she was harming her baby by taking her medication and also knew that if she stopped her medicine she would get severe anxiety and depression. Her obstetrician had referred her to a well-known geneticist, who explained the risks of taking medicine for anxiety and depression while pregnant. Her psychiatrist had already told her that the benefits of taking the medicine outweighed the risks for herself, and for her unborn baby.

Shana's doctor strongly recommended that she not change anything with her medication. He didn't think that she needed to consult a geneticist but went along with the idea, hoping that it might reassure Shana.

When Shana went to see the geneticist, the geneticist began the appointment by having her sign a lengthy release form that held the geneticist blameless if any harm came to Shana's unborn baby. This release form explained that she could still lose the baby, whether or not she took his advice, and that he was not responsible for any harm that might happen due to his advice. There were three pages of legal jargon explaining that there were no guarantees for a healthy pregnancy or a healthy baby.

Then he gave his advice. He explained about various studies, some of which were not even testing Shana's own medication, and explained how this might possibly mean that her medication was more dangerous than they realized. He also explained how there was still a percentage of chance for birth defects and that the "confidence interval" was acceptable.

He counseled her for an hour, summarized by saying that he could not tell her what to do, but that she could now make an informed decision, and then sent a report to her doctor explaining how the risks were within acceptable range for her to take her medication as prescribed.

If you're feeling anxious for Shana after reading this, then you can imagine how Shana felt when she walked out of this doctor's office. She was petrified and didn't even understand that this doctor was trying to tell her that she should take her medication throughout her pregnancy. When I spoke to the geneticist, he told me that he thought that Shana should continue her medication, but that is not the message that Shana understood. It took her psychiatrist and me quite a few sessions to help her understand that she and her baby were better off if she took her meds.

If your health care provider's use of jargon triggers your anxiety, be sure to ask them to explain your diagnosis and treatment in words you easily understand. Be willing to interrupt them and ask questions if what they say is difficult to understand. If they are unable to switch from using jargon to easy-to-understand language, then ask to speak with someone who can. Be willing to insist. You should not have to leave an appointment feeling confused about what your doctor or nurse thinks, what they prescribe, or why they are ordering tests or taking a wait-and-see approach.

Avoid the temptation to think that when a health care professional uses jargon it means they are smarter than you. It just means that they forgot to switch into everyday wording. Even complicated medical situations can be explained in easy-to-understand language. You need a doctor who makes it easy for you to avoid unnecessary anxiety, and who is willing to make sure you have an accurate understanding of your health care.

When Your Health Care System Is Afraid of Uncertainty

Some clinics and health care systems place a heavy emphasis on avoiding uncertainty, so they can decrease malpractice claims and avoid lawsuits. Hospitals and many larger clinics hire attorneys to help protect against malpractice, and develop policies to protect against frivolous claims, and against a patient failing to understand that no doctor can guarantee a good outcome, and no test can be 100 percent accurate.

Many doctors have had the misfortune of being sued for things outside of their control. This makes them rightly frightened about the possibility of future frivolous lawsuits. Unfortunately, the legally recommended procedure for minimizing the possibility of future frivolous malpractice claims is to have patients repeatedly sign lengthy release forms, and to have them follow a standard protocol for testing, even when it might not be medically necessary.

I have heard some doctors say, "If I were not at this hospital, I wouldn't have to order this test, but they want us to make sure that we overlook nothing, so no one gets sued. There was a doctor on staff who lost a lawsuit because the opposing attorney made the case that he should have ordered a repeat blood test. So now we have to do this second test."

Remember what happens when your mind takes a negative focus? If you have to read and sign release forms whenever you get a test or see a doctor, won't you start to wonder what could possibly go wrong? When you get that second test or second opinion, don't you start to get more anxious about the need for more tests and opinions? It just repeats the anxiety cycle all over again. This means that you're going to have to be savvy about what information you read and how you interpret the need for multiple release forms, more tests, and second opinions.

People who don't suffer from anxiety about illness usually don't bother to read or reread the release forms that are required each time you visit a health care provider. Why? They already know what these forms say and know that reading them wastes time and potentially makes them unnecessarily think about negative things that might happen. They realize that these forms are a required step for getting treatment but otherwise don't contribute to the likelihood of having a problem or of having something go wrong.

Unfortunately, if you're like many people with illness anxiety, reading these forms makes the odds of bad things happening seem more real, likely, and dangerous. If you keep rereading release forms, I suggest that you stop. You're making it harder to learn that seeking health care doesn't have to be a worrisome event. Make a commitment to yourself to avoid focusing upon negative things and what might go wrong. Sign your release forms, accepting that no doctor can guarantee a good outcome and that you don't need a guarantee in order to proceed with treatment. You may want to take a moment to reflect and write down what happens to your anxiety when you read release forms or get caught up in a medical system's desire to avoid lawsuits.

RAISING YOUR RESILIENCE: Write down a commitment to yourself to avoid letting your anxiety expect a perfect diagnosis or treatment. Write down your commitment to avoid reading all the fine print of release forms, and to reframe signing them as simply agreeing with the health care system that you give permission to be treated and there are no guarantees. Think of signing a release form as agreeing to a partnership with your health care team for everyone to do their best, including you, to ensure your good health. You can sign and date your own commitment to yourself.

When Your Doctor Believes in Giving You Reassurance

Health care professionals who don't understand the cycle of negative reinforcement and anxiety are likely to make the critical mistake of trying to give you more reassurance when they encounter your illness anxiety. They do this because they care and because they have not studied the modern treatment of anxiety. They do this because giving reassurance to patients who don't have illness anxiety works without any negative side effect. They also do this because their patients with illness anxiety reinforce giving reassurance, because they seek their doctor's reassurance and are very grateful for their reassurance. They may believe that giving you reassurance will make you feel better and make your anxiety go away, permanently.

I have known people with illness anxiety who specifically sought out a doctor because they knew that doctor had daily open hours when any patient could call in to ask their questions, even if the patient called several days every week. It feels good to your doctor or nurse when they help you feel calmer by providing reassurance, whether it's by convincing you that you're fine or ordering a test that gives you a normal result that they falsely believe will convince your anxious mind that you're okay. Often when I speak to these well-intentioned doctors, they tell me that they pride themselves in going the extra mile for their patients by providing extra reassurance—even though they can tell that it never really works when their patient has illness anxiety. They just don't understand how to best help.

You might wonder why your internist or pediatrician lacks information about treating illness anxiety. It's simple: most doctors and nurses who don't choose mental health as their specialty have only two to four weeks of clinical training in psychiatry prior to graduation. They might have heard about exposure therapy, but not had opportunities to see how to implement this type of treatment. They have probably been busy trying to study and keep up with the latest advances in their area of specialty. That is good news for your physical health, but makes it difficult for your doctor to address your mental health.

This is why it's incumbent upon you to take an honest look at how you interact with your health care team. Do you abuse the privilege of calling in, by calling to get rid of your anxiety instead of asking a necessary question? Do you take advantage of a well-intentioned health care provider by repeatedly asking "just one more question" in order to feel less anxious? Do you try to get your doctor to order more tests, instead of letting them make the decision or suggestion? Do you abuse the privilege of talking to the doctor when their office calls to say that your tests are normal/negative, just so you can hear someone confirm that everything is okay?

Andrew's Story

Andrew had a concierge doctor with a daily call-in hour, who also allowed his patients to text him with any questions. Andrew chose this doctor because he had a reputation for being kind, available, and for keeping the size of his practice small, so patients could always have easy access to him. Andrew, and all of the other patients in this doctor's practice, paid a special yearly fee so this doctor could maintain a small practice that allowed lots of doctor and patient interaction.

Whenever Andrew had his annual physical, he asked for multiple tests, to make sure that all of his body systems were in good health: blood tests, a urinalysis, and sometimes other tests. Before he got his tests, prior to each physical, Andrew would call the nurses to ask them what each test meant and to get their reassurance that all of his previous test results had been fine and that his future test results would be fine. He had several favorite nurses he would talk to, because they would remind Andrew of his doctor's expertise, experience, and ability to catch things early. These conversations made Andrew feel safer and less likely to get a bad result from his tests.

Once he arrived in the doctor's office for his annual physical, Andrew repeated the same reassurance-seeking conversation with the nurse who took his vital signs prior to seeing the doctor in person. He would ask the doctor to remind him that he was in good health and to explain what Andrew's chances were of getting cancer in the next year.

Following the in-person appointment, Andrew would call each day for the next one to two weeks, to get the doctor to re-explain his test results and the status of his health. Andrew would also ask the doctor about the accuracy of the tests, and on some occasions convinced the doctor to repeat the tests "just to be certain that everything was okay."

Do you now see how a well-intentioned doctor or nurse can accidentally make things worse while trying to make things better?

When to Seek Reassurance from Your Doctor

There are some occasions when it's appropriate to seek your doctor's reassurance, especially if you do have a serious health condition. In this instance, your doctor will need to confirm a serious diagnosis, order extra tests, speak to specialists, and provide realistic comfort about your treatment. The big difference in this case is that something is definitely wrong with your health. Illness anxiety always focuses on what *might* be wrong or what *might* go wrong.

It can take a while to adjust to a serious diagnosis and you'll need reminders and reassurance to help you make the adjustment. There will be a real problem to address and real treatments to receive. Part of your recovery will include addressing your illness anxiety, so you can focus on living as well as possible even though you might have a serious condition.

Have you ever let your anxiety drive you to take advantage of a health care provider's well-intentioned willingness to give you reassurance? Are you willing to give up this form of reassurance for the sake of your mental wellness and peace of mind? If you know that you have erred in this direction, you probably know that you need to stop taking advantage of your doctor's or nurses' willingness to reassure you, by explaining your illness anxiety and the problem that reassurance-seeking creates. You'll need to be willing to ask them to stop giving you inappropriate reassurance, and instead remind you that you seem to be struggling with anxiety.

RAISING YOUR RESILIENCE: Try to imagine what it would be like if you stopped trying to get reassurance or stopped asking for additional tests from your health care team. Write down your commitment to avoid accidentally letting your anxiety hijack your doctor's or nurse's kindness, and commit to never requesting their reassurance when nothing is wrong.

When Your Doctor Accidentally Cooperates with Your Avoidance

When doctors or clinics get busy, they can get into the practice of paying attention to only those patients who clamor for their attention. They can forget to follow up with patients who miss appointments, fail to get tests, or put off important screenings.

If your illness anxiety makes you put off getting tests, avoid seeing the doctor, or avoid getting necessary screenings, then you can get into trouble when your doctor or clinic fails to notice your absence. Avoidance not only makes your illness anxiety worse—it can have a negative effect on your health. You might end up like Tiffany.

Tiffany's Story

Tiffany had never seen a doctor since she graduated from high school thirty years ago. She came from a family with a history of diabetes, heart disease, thyroid disease, and early death. She was terrified of getting bad news from a doctor or nurse. She had good insurance and her workplace had a special arrangement where the insurance company would send out reminders to get annual physicals and screenings to anyone who had not done so.

She had actually made an appointment several years before meeting me but had been calling in every six months to "reschedule the appointment because I'm busy at work." She was registered with a doctor and had standing orders for blood tests, but had never met the doctor nor taken any tests. No one at the doctor's office asked her why she had been rescheduling for three years. They just kept rescheduling.

Tiffany completed therapy with me for her illness anxiety and had her first annual physical. Unfortunately, she learned that she did indeed have some significant health problems that needed treatment. Even though she was in treatment with me, the news of her health status made her start putting off her follow-up appointments with her internist, every week for two months. She hid her procrastination from me because she knew I would make her commit to an appointment. Once again, no one at her doctor's office asked her why she was rescheduling every week.

She would have put off her treatment indefinitely had I not asked more pointed questions about what she was doing to follow the doctor's recommendations. You can imagine what would have happened to her long-term health had she not been in treatment for her illness anxiety.

Overcoming Avoidance of Health Care

Do you secretly feel relieved when your health provider isn't paying attention? Do you avoid doctors or clinics who do pay close attention to how often you visit, or how rapidly you follow through with their recommendations? If so, then it's time for you to do some exposure practice by following through with appointments, screenings, and tests. Recognize that the longer you avoid, the more anxious you'll feel about making and keeping an appointment. Stop the cycle of negative reinforcement of your illness anxiety, by deciding that making and keeping your health care appointments is an important form of exposure practice. Remind yourself that like all exposure practice, making and keeping these important appointments will get easier the more you do it. Remember that the hardest part of exposure practice is usually deciding to do the practice and anticipating the practice, as opposed to the actual practice.

> **RAISING YOUR RESILIENCE:** Write down a list of the appointments, screenings, and tests that you have put off. Make a list of any excuses, such as "I'm too busy," "I cannot take time off from work," or "I couldn't bear the anxiety." Write down a personal statement that helps you remember how you're worth the effort to do what it takes to recover from illness anxiety. Don't let your anxiety about illness put your health in jeopardy.

Putting It All Together

What would your ideal health care team look like? It helps to know what you're looking for, so you can set up a health care team that works in favor of your physical *and* mental health. Even if you don't have a lot of choices about who you see because of your insurance, location, or health care system, you can still do things to help your health care team do their job in a manner tailored to your needs.

Most health care providers understand that many people suffer from anxiety and they have seen patients who have illness anxiety. They want to help you have the best mental and physical health possible, and they love it when you take charge of your health. They just need your help when they are not familiar with the treatments described in this book. Following are some suggestions that I have seen work well for people like you.

Inform your health care provider that you have illness anxiety. If they are not familiar with how illness anxiety can push you to seek reassurance and avoid tests or procedures, they are likely to misinterpret you as being uncooperative or not trusting their expertise and wisdom. They might even think that you don't want to work with them. Here is an example of how you could talk to your health care provider about your anxiety.

> "I would like you to know that I struggle with anxiety about serious illness. It can make me [describe what happens to you when you have an episode of illness anxiety]. Sometimes my anxiety can make me seek reassurance by repeatedly questioning my doctor, their staff, or going on the Internet to try and make sure I'm not seriously ill. This can happen no matter how much I trust you or your recommendations. I just get stuck wanting to make sure I'm not seriously ill.
>
> "I'm not a hypochondriac. I just get worries about illness stuck in my mind. I'm working on it, to try and not accidentally give in to asking too many questions and doing too much research.
>
> "It also makes me even more anxious when someone tells me to just stop worrying. I already know that! I just need your help to manage my anxiety, without accidentally making you or your staff misunderstand me."

Find a health care provider who is sympathetic to people with illness anxiety. Ask them how they feel about working with someone who accidentally gets anxious about illness. You could ask them like this:

> "How do you feel about working with people who have illness anxiety? What do you do when someone like me gets really anxious and needs more explanations or has a lot of questions?"

If your health care provider gives you a sympathetic response and tries to validate your anxiety, this is a good sign. If they seem to take your anxiety seriously, then you have found someone who is likely to be helpful.

Ask the nurses at your clinic, hospital, or doctor's office who they think is the best doctor or nurse for patients who get anxious about illness. Nurses often know best who has a kind way of working with patients and they will let you know.

Go online and look for reviews of your health care provider. Be careful and just look for the overall theme of the reviews, looking for a provider who is kind, patient, and willing to take the time to listen and respond to patient concerns. Ignore outlier negative reviews and look instead for the most frequent comments about how they work with people.

Feel empowered to switch health care providers if your experience with your doctor or nurse has been unhelpful. Sadly, some of my patients have told me about health care providers who have raised their voice, told them to leave the practice, or told them that they could not work with them if they continued reassurance-seeking. In each of these cases, the health care provider in question misunderstood the patient as lacking trust and confidence in the provider's care.

Take a support person who can encourage you to stick to your plan to avoid reassurance-seeking questions. Have your support person take notes if your anxiety makes it hard to listen, understand, and recall what your health care provider tells you. If you get flooded with anxiety when you're seeing a health care provider, having a supportive person to take notes can be truly helpful.

When you're ready, tell your health care provider that you would like their help in decreasing reassurance-seeking and avoidance. Help them help you by explaining to them how they can best be helpful. You can say it like this:

> "I'm following a plan to decrease the reassurance-seeking that maintains my anxiety about getting seriously ill, by trying not to

> ask extra questions. I could really use your help. Would you be willing to ask me if I'm getting anxious, if you notice I start asking repeat questions? Then, if I say 'yes,' you could say something like, 'Looks like you're really getting worried. I don't want to make it worse by accidentally giving you reassurance. How can I help you stay on track with your recovery right now? I know you'll feel better in the long run if I don't answer that question.'"

If you don't have a primary care doctor or nurse, get one. Try to use the same doctor and the same nurse whenever possible. Your goal is to develop a trusting relationship with your health care team. The two of you need to get to know and trust each other when you feel calm, which will make it easier for you to work together when you accidentally get anxious. It also is easier when your doctor and nurse know each other and work well together, so you know communication between them is good.

Creating a Healthy Partnership with Your Doctor

You should avoid using the emergency department unless it's a true emergency, as detailed in Chapter 6. Be willing to be assertive and call your primary care health team when you have genuine health concerns, so they get to know you well. This can prevent unnecessary testing and anxiety, because your team understands you. How can you tell when a health concern is something you should mention to your doctor? You will know when it is a genuine concern when the following circumstances are true:

- Non-anxious people with the same symptom would contact their doctor
- The symptom impairs your ability to do necessary tasks, such as go to work, do chores, and meet your daily responsibilities
- The symptom will not go away

- It is a symptom that your doctor, or a previous doctor, has told you to bring up to your doctor
- It is *not* one of the things that you typically get worried about

If something does not fit this list, then you can make a note to mention it to your doctor on your next regularly scheduled visit. It is important that you try not to let your anxiety determine when you contact your doctor, because this can make your illness anxiety worse. Instead, you want to create a system of regularly scheduled health screenings and physical exams, so your doctor gets to know you and your body well. This will increase your ability to trust their judgment and to work cooperatively with them, especially when you also disclose that you get anxious and worry about illness.

If you tend to only use the walk-in or urgent care clinic, then you'll never have the experience of working with someone who understands your illness anxiety. You risk having someone either dismiss your concerns when nothing is wrong, or over-respond to your concerns in an effort to do a good job, without recognizing the negative effect this can have on your anxiety.

Clinics are designed to look for emergencies and urgent issues, and are therefore more likely to think about and order tests for more serious health concerns, which might not be necessary and could make your anxiety worse.

Start getting an annual physical, if you don't already. Don't let your anxiety dictate when you get health care or preventive health care. You need a health care team that does the recommended screenings and assessments that are best for your long-term health. Having annual health information on hand makes it much easier for your doctor or nurse to speak with authority about the status of your health and your individual health risks. They can better advise you on your lifestyle, medications, and recommended precautions than when you only see them for occasional health concerns, or when your anxiety is triggered. Many people with illness anxiety procrastinate scheduling annual physicals because they fear getting bad news. But this increases anxiety and puts your health at risk.

Set up regular check-ins with your health care team, for any chronic conditions that require ongoing treatment. Don't wait to let your anxiety set the schedule. Follow the schedule for the treatment and evaluation your health care provider suggests and stick to it.

Save your questions for your doctor or nurse until the next scheduled appointment. This is what people who are not anxious about their health do. If you have an acute illness or something that meets the standard for requiring immediate attention, then please do contact your health care team—but otherwise, keep a list of things you want to discuss and save it for your annual physical or the next time you visit your doctor. Avoid the temptation to call, text, or email each time your anxiety gives rise to a question, so you can get out of the habit of reassurance-seeking. Questions you should save for the next visit are about your long-term health status, your personal risk factors, the treatment plan going forward (if the current one doesn't work), or any new information about your health, your medications, or your personal risk factors.

Suggest your doctor or nurse read this book. Explain to them that this could help them better understand you and learn to be more effective in helping you. Offer to give them a copy or photocopy some parts of the book that you think would be especially helpful. Many health care professionals would be delighted to learn more but just need some guidance on what to read.

What You Have Learned

By this point, you should have a clear understanding of what happens when you get anxious. You should also be aware of some skills and practices that will help you overcome your illness anxiety, including the following:

- knowing the difference between the false alarm of anxiety and a real health emergency
- exposure to thoughts, sensations, and situations that make you anxious
- decreasing or stopping reassurance-seeking
- decreasing or avoiding anxiety-triggering situations
- coaching your support people to avoid giving you reassurance when you slip
- reframing your worries and anxiety episodes as reminders that the real problem is your anxiety, not the content of what you're worrying about
- reframing your anxiety and worry as opportunities to practice coping
- enlisting the help of your health care team and supportive friends and family

The skills described in Chapters 1 through 8 are science-proven strategies that will help you gain the upper hand in overcoming your illness anxiety. The next chapter offers something different: the opportunity to learn skills from the field of positive psychology (the study of what creates mental wellness), which recent research has shown prevents anxiety and helps people who have anxiety become more resilient and able to enjoy their lives.

The fun thing about learning the skills in Chapter 9 is that none of them involve facing your fears! And if you practice them, you'll find they rapidly help you feel better about who you are and what you're doing, even when you're anxious.

CHAPTER 9

Express Gratitude to Build Joy and Resilience

What would you say if I told you there's something that you can write down each day for the next thirty days that could improve your mental and physical health? It would only take five to seven minutes a day and you would not have to see a therapist or join a support group. You would probably be begging me to hurry up and tell you which words to write down!

Well, here it is: the words you need to write down are words of gratitude. That's it! It's so simple. If you want to improve your mental and physical health over the next thirty days, you need to start writing down the things that you realize are an undeserved blessing for which you can be grateful.

I know that it sounds preposterous, but there's a large body of science—more than fifteen thousand studies, to be exact—studying the powerful effect gratitude has on mental and physical health (Tala 2019). Science proves when you make the time to identify, articulate, and savor what you're grateful for each day, then you have the mental and physical health advantage over those who don't (Allen 2018).

What Is Gratitude?

Gratitude is your ability to perceive that something good or positive has occurred and to recognize that it's a blessing that's not a product of your own doing (Emmons and McCullough 2003). When someone feels grateful, they realize that what they experience is a gift, one that cannot be bought, earned, or produced. For example, when you take your first sip of coffee, tea, or orange juice in the morning, do you take a moment to consider how fortunate you are to be able to purchase the ingredients for your morning drink? Do you think about what it took to grow and harvest the things that went into your beverage? Do you think how fortunate you are to be able to taste and smell your beverage, to notice that you're alive and able to have this experience? This is gratitude.

This grateful focus is much more than counting your blessings. It's savoring the blessing of being alive and able to experience something good, no matter how small or seemingly insignificant. It's the ability to find and acknowledge the beauty of the moment.

Gratitude is not just what you feel and think when things are going well. It can occur at any moment and in any circumstance, including in the middle of suffering. For example, if you're in an automobile accident, you can realize that you're alive, that the ambulance is nearby, and that there are doctors who will do their best to help you recover. You can be grateful that your body always attempts to heal itself when it's injured. You can be grateful that you didn't suffer a more disabling injury.

If you're really skilled at gratitude, you can experience a severe panic attack and several days of lost sleep after getting triggered and still find the blessing in being able to read this book—to be alive and on the path to recovery. You might even be grateful for the examples of real people in this book, who give you hope because they recovered from their illness anxiety.

The most important gratitude is often the gratitude you feel when life is difficult or when painful circumstances enter your life. Gratitude reminds you that no matter how bad things may seem, there's still goodness, blessings, and hope until your very last breath.

That may seem like an impossible challenge when illness anxiety is focused on every terrible thing that might occur. Gratitude, however, is a worthy challenge for you to undertake, precisely *because* your anxiety repeatedly pushes you to think about the worst and to contemplate the awful.

Do you want to be the anxious person who overlooked the hundreds of daily blessings in your life, or do you want to be the anxious person who saw the beauty and joy of your daily life? What is really terrific about incorporating the practice of gratitude into your daily life is that the more you focus on gratitude, the harder it will be for your anxiety to destroy your healthy perspective on life.

You might be reacting to the idea of gratitude with cynicism. This is understandable. Modern western culture idealizes skepticism and cynicism, because they give the illusion of being smart (Stavrova and Ehlenbracht 2018). If you're cynical, then you might believe that you can protect yourself from disappointment by anticipating a negative event ahead of time.

Unfortunately, by doing so, you also protect yourself from good mental health. You end up wasting the good moments of your life on feeling the dread of imagined illness or on the thought of dying miserably when nothing has yet happened. Do you really want to spend your good days feeling the pain of imagined bad days?

Furthermore, if you try to avoid or suppress one emotion, such as disappointment or anxiety, then you accidentally risk suppressing any emotion, including positive ones. You need to allow yourself to experience the full range of emotions, even when some of them are unpleasant.

Part of being emotionally mature entails feeling many emotions at once. For example, you might feel sad when you hear about a friend's bad news, while simultaneously feeling frustrated at not finding a parking space *and* feeling excited about getting a raise in your paycheck. You feel all three things at the same time, without compromising your ability to function or notice the emotion associated with each experience.

This ability to feel the full range of emotion makes it possible to dull the sharpness of painful emotions and to restore hope after being disappointed or hurt. It also helps you realize that each emotion is ephemeral. When you understand this, it makes it easier to feel gratitude for all the little blessings of your day. You stop taking happiness and blessings for granted. Gratitude also gives you the ability to remain in touch with what is good, even when things feel very painful. Gratitude improves your ability to experience these blended emotions in a beneficial way.

Health Benefits of Gratitude

When you feel gratitude, you release a host of feel-good, healing chemicals into your body, which elevate your mood, decrease inflammation, and restore your body to a healthy resting state (Millstein et al. 2016, Sirois and Wood 2016.) These physiological changes help you recover from the experience of feeling anxious and help you reset your body to a non-anxious state.

This is very important if you have had illness anxiety for longer than a few months. Your body likely needs help learning how to return to a full resting state, instead of constantly being on high alert. When you practice gratitude, you recover from serious illness more rapidly, can prevent chronic illness, and are more likely to follow through with good health behaviors (Emmons and McCullough 2003, Krause et al. 2017). You can improve your sleep and decrease insomnia by practicing gratitude (M.-Y. Ng and Wong 2013). This can be really helpful, because if you're like most people with anxiety, you know that your sleep gets disrupted when you're anxious.

Krause et al. (2017) found that stronger levels of gratitude lower blood markers associated with diabetes, heart disease, several cancers, and kidney failure. People who are habitually grateful also develop fewer illnesses, have lower blood pressure, and live an average of seven years longer than people who have the same health-risk factors but are not regularly practicing gratitude (Randolph 2017, APA 2020). So if you care about your physical health, you'll want to learn how to practice gratitude.

The Mental Health Benefits of Gratitude

Gratitude is not just good for your physical health. It's really important for your mental health. When you have a grateful mindset, you'll be happier, more optimistic (which is a predictor of resilience, persistence, and success), earn better grades, and make more money than people who are just like you but are not skilled at practicing gratitude. If you're grateful each day, then you'll be happier in your relationships, and your partners, family, and friends will be happier and more pleased with you (Randolph 2017, APA 2020).

If you're willing to track your gratitude, you'll also be more likely to experience improved relationships with your friends and family, because you'll begin to notice their thoughtfulness and kindness that you used to overlook (Williams and Bartlett 2014). When you practice gratitude, you're more likely to express appreciation, which is priceless for maintaining a healthy relationship. In other words, gratitude makes you more likeable.

If you experience a trauma and you're regularly practicing gratitude, you'll recover better and faster than someone who doesn't. Lastly, when you practice gratitude, *you'll have lower levels of anxiety and depression* (Randolph 2017, APA 2020).

An attitude of gratitude also motivates you to help others and prevents unhealthy personality characteristics from developing, such as envy, entitlement, narcissism, cynicism, and materialism (Algoe, Gable, and Maisel 2010). Envy happens when you devalue who you are and what you have in relation to someone else. Entitlement is the belief that good things are your birthright and deprivation from privilege is an insult. Narcissism occurs when you're unable to care about someone else's emotions and believe that the only way to feel good in life is to be admired and praised, even without having earned the right to be admired or praised. Cynicism is the assumption that no person, institution, or circumstance can be trusted, because everyone will operate out of selfish self-interest and ignore the greater good. Materialism is valuing things and status over relationships.

You can see why you would want to avoid this list of toxic characteristics. They are markers of poor mental health and distressed or broken relationships. They inhibit your path to joy, good relationships, and self-worth.

When you practice gratitude, you develop humility, which is the ability to recognize that you're simply a human being like everyone else, simultaneously flawed and frustrated with being flawed. You feel comfortable not being "all that," even if you hold a title or an award that suggests otherwise. You don't require praise or admiration in order to feel full of worth and purpose. You don't need for things to go your way in order to be happy, whether it's an anxiety-free day, a perfect report of good health from the doctor, or avoiding tragedy. You start to realize that each day of life is a precious gift to be savored.

When you become humble, you lose your sense of shame about being an anxious person and you recognize that you're not alone in your suffering. Your humility, in turn, makes it easier to experience even more gratitude, because you begin to perceive the hundreds of daily moments of blessing that are part of your life even when you suffer.

So, you can see that gratitude has much to offer you. If you want to move past envy of those who are not anxious, or shame about being anxious, or overcome the negative mental preset of an anxious mind, then you'll want to pay close attention to what follows in this chapter.

Let me tell you about the story of Janice.

Janice's Story

Janice came to see me when her family encouraged her to get help for her illness anxiety. Her grown children and husband told her that she was really negative, and always thinking about the worst-case scenario, even though nothing bad had ever happened to her or her family. Her husband, especially, told her that he "could not stand to hear another negative thing from her mouth" and threatened to move out if she didn't change soon. He told her that he would not divorce her, but he feared for his own mental health if he had to hear more worry about terrible illnesses and other bad things.

Janice told me, "I know I shouldn't do it, but I just keep feeling like I live under a rain cloud and that something terrible is always about to happen. I know my life is good and everyone is healthy thus far, but what if everything goes wrong tomorrow?"

Janice quickly began working on her illness anxiety. She stopped researching terrible illnesses, stopped checking her and her family's health symptoms, began avoiding conversations about other people's illnesses, and began doing exposure practice to scary words, serious illnesses, and the thought of dying. She made some good initial progress and impressed her family and friends by no longer drawing the conversation toward reassurance-seeking. She was even able to watch medical TV shows without going into a panic.

She then told me, "I know that I'm doing the best that I have ever done since I started worrying about getting sick, but I still just don't feel happy and healthy. I wake up every day feeling like this is the day that something terrible will happen. It's like a habit that my gut just assumes that something bad is about to happen."

This is when I introduced the idea of practicing gratitude to Janice, explaining to her how the negative focus of her anxiety had made it difficult for her to learn how to notice what was good, what was a blessing, and even what felt good each day. She took on the thirty-day challenge to write down three things every day that she recognized were good and positive, a blessing derived from something outside of herself. For example, feeling a sense of accomplishment is nice when you finish knitting a hat, but feeling grateful for the sheep that produced the wool, or feeling grateful to your ancestors who gifted you the genetics for good hand-eye coordination, is gratitude. I told Janice to force herself to write down three things she was grateful for each day, even if she was feeling anxious or panicky.

It was difficult for Janice to find things to write down the first several days, because she had always made the mistake of thinking that she needed to feel free of anxiety in order to notice or feel a positive emotion such as gratitude. Once she had several days recorded in her journal, however, it became easier and more fun. She actually started feeling gratitude while she was writing, and when she recalled what she had written. After a week, she even had a day in which she wrote more than three things. After two weeks, she noticed that she was keeping track of things to write down in her journal and this felt fun and uplifting. She noticed that she could feel full of gratitude even when she still felt some anxiety.

By week three, she told me, "I just feel happier and like my life is better. I think I was always feeling sorry for myself because of my anxiety and because I always felt like something terrible was going to happen."

By the end of thirty days, she told me that she wanted to keep a gratitude journal for the rest of her life because it made her feel so much better. She had even told her husband and children about her gratitude challenge and suggested they try it for themselves.

RAISING YOUR RESILIENCE: Take a moment to reflect upon the emotional price you pay for trying to avoid your anxiety and for taking a negative view of your life. Write down the emotional cost you have paid from slipping into cynicism, or into a negative worldview. If you want to live a full, zesty life, then you have to allow yourself the full range of emotions, including anxiety and disappointment. Be willing to build up your ability to appreciate the contrast between gratitude for every little blessing and your negative, anxious view of life. The good things will feel that much sweeter.

Gratitude and Persistence

Gratitude also improves your ability to be persistent (Williams and Bartlett 2014). This is really important to your recovery. You need to be willing to practice your exposure and challenge your unhelpful thoughts and beliefs until it becomes habit —and even when it feels really difficult. This requires great persistence. Refining your ability to feel gratitude will give you the strength and desire to pick yourself up when your worry or anxiety seems too much, because you know that blessings will be ahead.

Allen's Story

Allen had seen many therapists before he met me. He introduced himself as a hopeless case and informed me that I was his last attempt at therapy, and then he would give up once he failed with me. He told me that he thought I would only last a few sessions until I fired him from treatment because his case was so hopeless.

Instead of diving into exposure-based exercises, I decided to help Allen tackle his demoralized view of himself. I assigned him the thirty-day gratitude challenge several weeks after we started working together. He thought the exercise was silly and inauthentic, because his suffering was so chronic and disabling. He believed that he would be one of my worst patients ever and that there was nothing to feel grateful for, because he always felt riddled with anxiety.

I told him to write down things that were real, and to write down three things no matter how he felt, even if it was something like "I'm glad that someone figured out how to flavor my toothpaste, so it tastes better," or "I'm glad that my pants have a zipper that works so I don't have to button my pants." He told me, "This sounds so trite. I would feel grateful if someone would find a cure for my anxiety. Now that's gratitude!"

But Allen told me that once he started, he found that he could actually find three things to write down, which surprised him. He had to work hard to find three things to write in his journal, and it took him all day to find three things, but they were real things. He wrote about having a house to live in and having a dog who always enjoyed being near him, even when he was irritable and anxious.

He kept at it and, after several weeks, he began writing down more than three things. He started noticing lots of things that made him feel grateful, such as how comfortable his desk chair was, how much he liked being able to ride the train to work instead of having to drive, or how blessed he was to not have dentures.

Then he noticed that it was becoming easier to recover from unexpected triggers to his anxiety, instead of getting severely disappointed and thinking, Here I go again. One step forward and four steps back. His inner self-talk became, instead, I really am recovering. I'm moving forward. I just have to pick myself up and keep trying. This time I'm really going to succeed, because I'm never going to give up. I'm so glad that I didn't give up.

How Grateful Are You?

Have you ever taken the time to assess how easily you feel gratitude each day? Take some time to reflect on these questions and identify areas that you need to address, in order to improve your ability to experience gratitude. Write down reminders to yourself to pay attention to the areas in which you realize you fall short.

Do you readily:

- Take delight in the goodness of others?
- Find and take delight in the beauty around you in nature?
- Delight in the privileges and blessings of your day or life?
- Feel grateful for your heritage, culture, and ancestors?
- Experience gratitude for the blessing of being alive?
- Feel grateful for the people in your life?
- Feel grateful for the experiences of your day?
- Feel grateful for the things you have learned?
- Feel grateful for the material blessings of your life? Your clothing? Food? Shelter? Opportunities? Education? Vacations? Hobbies? Books? Digital devices?
- Feel grateful for the blessings that good people bestow on others?
- Feel grateful for the divine in your life, such as God, love, or the spiritual power(s) in the universe?

You can compare your ability to feel gratitude to other people's by taking the Gratitude Quiz at https://greatergood.berkeley.edu/quizzes/take_quiz/gratitude.

How to Practice Gratitude

Savoring is an important part of practicing gratitude. When writing down what you're grateful for, just writing a long list of single-word items or rapidly rushing through a list of stock answers doesn't work. This is why, even though you may pray prayers of gratitude, such as saying grace before meals or thanking God in a worship service, you might not have cultivated gratitude.

In order to cultivate gratitude, you have to *focus on something that is meaningful to you and identify what about this experience is a blessing.* Research shows that the more you savor your gratitude, the better it works (Pitts 2018). Thus, writing down a description of what happened, how you felt, and why you felt that way works better than just writing down a one- or two-word representation of the moment. Writing longhand works better than typing, possibly because you have more time to savor the experience. If you're keeping a diary or journal, stick to things that happened in the last twenty-four hours, and force yourself to find three things. Sharing what you're grateful for aloud, and explaining it to others, also helps you savor your blessings. Here is an example of a helpful and unhelpful gratitude journal entry.

> *Helpful:* I'm so glad that I could order a desk lamp in this pretty shade of blue. It makes me happy to see how it coordinates with the other fun colors in my office. It makes it fun to look at my desk. I'm so glad that I have the money to be able to order a lamp like this.
>
> *Unhelpful:* Blue desk lamp

Saving your gratitude lists allows you to go back and reread experiences to savor again and again. Past journals can inspire you when you're feeling anxious or discouraged.

In 2006, I began my daily gratitude practice, which continues to this day. I hope that you'll join me in cultivating a lifestyle of gratitude.

I have years of saved journals. I keep them on a shelf next to my desk, so I can reread them when I have a rough day or feel low in motivation. I also take a moment to practice gratitude prior to doing difficult tasks, because I know that it recharges my mental and emotional batteries. This is why I want my past gratitude journals close by. When you reread your gratitude journals, you can get double the effect, because you'll reexperience the gratitude from when you first wrote about it in your journal.

RAISE YOUR RESILIENCE: Consider using sturdy and attractive notebooks to record your gratitude, so you can store them for the future. Having an attractive journal honors the significance of your moments of gratitude. Be willing to read through past records of gratitude and regard them as evidence of priceless emotional jewels.

Creating a Lifestyle of Gratitude

Initially, it helps to practice gratitude every day for the first month, to help create the habit and to develop your ability to perceive the blessings of your life. After the first month, it helps to record your gratitude about three times per week, so it doesn't become a chore (Allen 2018).

Recording gratitude is an important part of the practice of gratitude, but there's more. Your goal is to be able to find things to be grateful for at any moment on any day of your life. This means taking the time to mindfully notice what is going on during your day, instead of rushing through it. The practice of gratitude implies that you make room for observing and savoring each blessing as it comes your way. This takes time.

See if you can learn to think of noticing your blessings in the moment as having the same significance as drinking water or eating food. It's nourishment for your heart and soul. Avoid the temptation to become focused on being too busy, so you accidentally treat your practice of gratitude as another thing to check off your to-do list. This defeats the purpose.

RAISE YOUR RESILIENCE: Overcome the temptation to put off cultivating a lifestyle of gratitude. Knowing the value of gratitude is not the same as practicing gratitude. Be intentional about making gratitude a regular part of your life. If you have mental obstacles to taking the time to become a habitually grateful person, take a moment to pause and think about them. Does it feel like another chore to have to start a gratitude journal? Take a moment to gentle your breathing and quiet your mind, to imagine what it would feel like to make room for gratitude. What might happen in your life if you allowed yourself the time to notice and feel blessings in your life every day? Would you feel more peaceful, energized, or more refreshed and able to live in your skin?

Sharing Gratitude

The practice of gratitude also involves sharing gratitude. When you learn to slow down and settle into your awareness of what blesses you, you naturally begin to want to share this with others. When you share your gratitude with others, you inspire them to experience gratitude, which blesses them. When you readily express appreciation to others, you revitalize your relationships, whether it's at work or at home.

If you have ever been around someone who readily experiences and expresses gratitude, you know how good it feels to hear them say, "I'm so glad you just walked in. I love seeing your smile." You know how encouraging it feels to be told, "That is such a great idea. It will make this project so much better."

Your expression of gratitude is so important because it inspires trust, hope, and cooperation. It makes people want to be around you and to reciprocate your expressions of gratitude. So, be willing to speak aloud your gratitude, whether it's about that person, the situation, or just something you noticed. For example, how great might it feel if someone walked into work and announced, "Hey, guess what happened to me today? Someone in line in front of me paid for my coffee." Chances are you and your coworkers would start talking about random acts of kindness and feel happier. Contrast this with the typical comment someone makes when they enter the office: "I cannot believe how bad the traffic was on the way into work." Giving voice to daily blessings you notice helps everyone who hears you appreciate the wonder and blessing of being alive together. You lift each other up.

> **RAISING YOUR RESILIENCE:** How do you feel about letting others know about your gratitude for their presence in your life and for what you experience in your day? Do you feel uncomfortable or foolish about sharing your moments of gratitude? Do you feel shy? Try to identify if an unhelpful belief or cultural message about skepticism and cynicism might be the obstacle. Write this down in your journal or notebook and state your commitment to prioritize your gratitude and joy over whatever might be getting in the way. Make it your goal to share gratitude with the people around you, so you can multiply joy in yourself and others.

EXERCISE The Thirty-Day Gratitude Challenge

1. Create or find a nice journal or notebook for recording your experiences of gratitude. You can download a gratitude practice sheet here: www.newharbinger.com/49043.
2. Select a time each day to reflect on your day and identify three things for which you are grateful. If you're a morning person, first thing in the morning might work well. Conversely if you're an evening person, recording your gratitude before bedtime might be better. Make a commitment to yourself to spend five to seven minutes each day to record three things for which you're grateful.
3. Avoid the temptation to record things you checked off your to-do list or things that are an accomplishment, unless you're focusing on what these experiences taught or revealed to you about being blessed. Write down things that create a feeling of

being blessed, being delighted, or being a humble recipient of something good.

4. Write down what happened, what gives you the feeling of delight, and what about it makes you grateful. Here are some examples:
   - How my orchid keeps blooming month after month even though I'm not a plant person. It has the perfect shade of purple that makes me smile.
   - My son's loud laughter and how it rolls out and he cannot stop and it makes the rest of us laugh too.
   - The view outside my office: being able to see green trees, the pond, and the Canadian geese.
   - How comfy my favorite sweats feel and being able to hang out in them all day.
   - Being done with mowing the lawn so I can rest and enjoy the yard in my hammock for the remainder of the day.
   - My partner cooking dinner and putting away laundry. Makes me feel so loved and freed from chores after a long day's work.
5. Make yourself write down three things each day, no matter how much your illness anxiety gets in the way. It's especially important to stick to your plan when you struggle, because it will help lift your mood and inspire you to persevere even when your day feels difficult. You'll discover that there's still good in the midst of anxiety.

EXERCISE The Thirty-Day Gratitude-Sharing Challenge—With One Person

1. Identify one person to share your gratitude with, every day for thirty days. Commit to letting them know which blessings you have experienced that day and describing what about the

situation or experience was a blessing. Ask that person to do the same with you, to be willing to share 1–3 things that they experienced as blessings for that day. You can do this by text, email, in person, over the phone or video conference, or a combination of these—whatever allows you to have a conversation with each other about experiencing gratitude.

2. Be sure to express gratitude each day to this person for listening and sharing their gratitude with you!

EXERCISE The Thirty-Day Gratitude-Sharing Challenge—With Many People

1. This challenge should be attempted after you do the one-person challenge. This challenge helps you build joy in your community of family, friends, and colleagues.
2. On day one, express your gratitude about a person's presence in your life to that one person. For example, when you say "Good morning" to your child, express your gratitude by saying something like, "Good morning. I'm so glad that you're my kid. You help to remind me that life is an adventure to be explored, with all of your ideas of what to do." Or to your friend, "I'm so glad you're my friend. You have always been so patient and kind when I'm having a rough day, and so faithful at replying to me when I need your help."
3. On day two, express your gratitude to two people.
4. On day three, express your gratitude to three people, and to four people on the fourth day, etc.—until you're expressing your gratitude to thirty people on day thirty.
5. If you don't encounter in your daily life the number of friends/family/coworkers corresponding to the number of the challenge day, aim to express gratitude to those people who are part of your day. This means paying attention to the grocery

clerk, the security guard, the customer service person who replied to your email, etc.—everyone you encounter. Your goal is to become really proficient at noticing all the blessings that other people provide in your life every day.

Radical Gratitude

If you want to get radically good at gratitude, then I have an even bigger challenge for you. It involves recognizing the blessing that is yours because of your anxiety about illness and dying.

When you learn to find the blessings that come from struggle and suffering, you acquire advanced emotional skills that can help you flourish throughout your life (Kreitzer et al. 2019). People who recover best from trauma and tragedy view their painful experiences as a priceless life lesson. They say things like, "I would never wish anxiety on anyone, but because of my anxiety, I have learned to be so much more compassionate and patient than I ever could have otherwise." They take themselves out of the self-pity zone of feeling like a victim of anxiety, and view their suffering as the crucible that formed their better self. They view themselves as a heroic person in their adventure of life, instead of as a tragic victim of anxiety.

The hero's journey, as you likely know from literature, involves a central character on an epic journey. The central character meets many challenges that reveal a personal flaw or vulnerability that impedes their journey and results in a painful loss or defeat. The heroic central character then learns to master the flaw or overcome their vulnerability, to become their better self who triumphs on their journey. It takes guts to transform your personal narrative of yourself from tragic into heroic.

What would happen if you took a heroic perspective about your anxiety? Wouldn't you rather be on an epic adventure of learning to live with your anxiety while becoming your better self? You really can learn to perceive and feel the blessings of being an anxious person when you take the time to discover what your experience is teaching you about what it means to be human and to suffer. Your anxious suffering doesn't have to be wasted pain. Your anxious suffering only becomes meaningless when you give in to self-pity and victimhood.

Victimhood is the opposite of a resilient, heroic mindset. When you view yourself as a victim of your anxiety, you accidentally assume the mindset of a tragic person who lacks dignity and hope. You assume that you're powerless, helpless, and have no options for how you think and act. You become passive and view yourself with pity, because you're dependent on the mercy of fate or of other more capable and powerful people. You forget that one of the innate strengths of human beings is the ability to learn, adapt, and grow throughout the entire lifespan, including when you're anxious.

When you align with a victim mindset, you settle for less by taking the anxious person's stance of "better safe than sorry," and don't take any risks. You give up the opportunity to become more capable, stronger, and more resilient. You prevent yourself from experiencing the joy that comes from struggling to find the blessing that is in your life and the experience of knowing you're capable of heroic struggle that leads to better things.

Gratitude can give you the inner strength to keep trying when you feel you have failed, or when you feel beset by anxiety. When you dig deep and search for the important life lessons that your anxiety can teach you, you discover that your fear can teach you many important things that can only be acquired by learning to strive though anxious moments.

Christine's Story

Christine is an example of someone who was determined to learn radical gratitude and dig herself out of chronic self-pity and cynicism, by reflecting upon what her anxiety was teaching her. She had illness anxiety for more than forty years before she met me. Her family was fed up with her anxiety and reassurance-seeking. She knew that they didn't respect her and only tolerated her because they felt a familial duty to not abandon her.

Christine felt like a total failure at life and could not recall any happy times from her past. She took the three previously mentioned thirty-day gratitude challenges, one month at a time. After these three months of challenges, she began journaling about what her experience of illness anxiety had taught her and was teaching her. Here is a sample of her list.

- *Anxiety has taught me to be compassionate toward myself and toward other people who have mental health problems. I used to feel sorry for people who saw therapists. Now I realize that they are good people who are just like everyone else.*
- *I have learned that everyone has problems of some kind and no one escapes suffering. Mine just happens to be anxiety.*
- *I'm much more patient with myself and other people. I have learned that some things are easy to learn and no big achievement, and some things are hard to learn, and those things are the biggest achievements.*
- *It's okay that life is not fair. I'm glad that I only have to deal with anxiety, instead of a lifetime of abuse.*
- *I'm braver and more capable than I ever believed possible.*
- *I have learned how to be persistent and struggle while being well.*
- *I can be full of joy even when I know that my anxiety could get triggered by some unexpected trigger.*
- *I'm no longer willing to settle for a stunted life. I'm willing to make things happen in my life and that means everything to me.*
- *I'm no longer angry and resentful toward my family for how they treated me. I was really difficult to live with and they were doing the best they could. I wore them out along*

with wearing myself out. No wonder they were fed up. I'm just so glad that we get along so much better and that they didn't give up on me and kick me out of their lives.

- *I now know how I can make other people happy, by sharing my gratitude. I don't have to just give them presents and hope they are not annoyed.*

As you can see from Christine's list, she has thought deeply about how anxiety has shaped her life in a good way, a way that really matters to her. She was willing to look past the disappointment of having to live with anxiety and to find the deeper meaning behind her suffering and her struggle to grapple with her suffering. She even began to think about taking on new hobbies and making new friends outside her small, safe circle of comfort. This took courage, for her to buck the culture of perfectionism, and the cultural definition of success that doesn't allow visible failure, such as a lifetime of being crippled by anxiety.

Christine realized that when success comes easily, it's not as meaningful as when someone has to struggle and overcome defeat in order to reach the same goal. This is why we are moved by the story of a combat veteran who learns to walk and run after losing several limbs in battle. It's why we love the story of the apparent loser or nerd who ends up saving the planet.

We all realize that, deep inside, we each have limitations that make some things difficult to attain. When you're honest with yourself about your limitations, you develop humility and realize that your greatest strengths will develop only when they are refined through your life struggles.

This is the value of learning to be radically grateful. This is the reason that you should hope to tell yourself, "I would not wish my anxiety on anyone, but I know without a doubt that I would not be the strong, capable, and good person that I am today had it not been for my struggle with anxiety. If I could live my life again, I would not change this part of my life, because I could not be who I am without it."

RAISE YOUR RESILIENCE: Be willing to challenge your unhelpful belief that your life could only be good if you never had another episode of anxiety. Instead, work hard to know that your life is beautiful and full of blessings, *because* your anxiety gave you the opportunity to develop great courage, compassion, and strength. Take a moment to write down in your journal or notebook what you hope to learn from your experience of illness anxiety.

Exercises to Help You Develop Radical Gratitude

The following activities are options for building your gratitude muscle. You can pick and choose, do any or all. You might find that you need to start with whichever exercise feels easiest to you and work up to the more challenging ones. There is no right order. What matters is that you attempt to broaden your perspective on what you stand to gain from living a life that includes anxiety and living in a vulnerable human body.

EXERCISE Gratitude Exercise 1

Write down your answers to the following questions and discuss the answers with people whom you know to be compassionate and validating of your experience.

1. What do you understand about yourself and your ability to be compassionate because of your anxiety?
2. Are there situations or people you now view differently because of your anxiety?
3. What skills are you developing because of your anxiety?
4. What skills have you had to strengthen because of your anxiety?

5. What has happened to your ability to be humble because of your anxiety?
6. What do you *not* take for granted, that others take for granted, because of your anxiety?
7. Are there ways that you're more helpful to others because of your anxiety?
8. What things are you more accepting of in yourself and others because of your anxiety?
9. What attitudes do you have about mental illness and treatment because of your anxiety that you might not otherwise have understood?
10. What are you able to give to society or to others because of your anxiety?

EXERCISE Gratitude Exercise 2

Read memoirs or biographies of people who have had to overcome mental illness, disability, grave injuries, trauma, or tragedy. Compare your experience to theirs and listen carefully to what they believe they have learned from their suffering. Try on their attitudes about very difficult life experiences.

EXERCISE Gratitude Exercise 3

Watch TED talks from speakers who have overcome great personal tragedy or abuse. Listen carefully to what they have learned and how they think about their own suffering and their purpose in life.

EXERCISE Gratitude Exercise 4

Practice radical gratitude daily, by pushing yourself to identify what is good about a painful experience while you're in the middle of it.

EXERCISE Gratitude Exercise 5

Interview someone who practices radical gratitude even though they have experienced tragedy or health challenges. If you are not sure how to find someone like this, ask a nurse who works in hospice if they know someone who is full of joy, love, and gratitude even though they are dying. Then ask the person what they have learned through their suffering and what makes them grateful about being alive.

My Story

When I had a bowel perforation that led to sepsis and nearly died several years ago, I was overwhelmed with the lengthy recovery, which involved having an ostomy bag (a bag attached to my belly that collected the contents of my small bowel), having an open incision that went from my bikini line to my sternum, and having to be on a constant intravenous line for six months. I was full of horror when I looked at my gaping incision, my ostomy bag, and my gray complexion. I was weak and in constant pain. I knew that I was anxious, sad, full of self-pity, and impatient to recover but powerless to speed up the process of recovery.

However, I knew that I didn't want to be depressed, anxious, and feeling sorry for myself, so I forced myself to write in my gratitude journal each day. I also forced myself to express my gratitude to my husband and home nurse, even though their care involved a lot of lengthy and painful procedures.

I also reminded myself that somehow, some way, I was going to learn something from this experience that would be of great benefit to my patients, family, and friends. I was not going to let my suffering go to waste! Even though I didn't know how I would get through it, I knew that I was going to somehow survive and thrive by learning something valuable. I wanted to someday look back on those difficult and painful days with gratitude.

Just being able to restate my commitment to future growth gave me hope and kept me from giving in to despair. It also kept me on the lookout for what was good about each day, because I knew that a blessing was present if only I would allow myself to perceive it. I knew that my biggest challenge was my attitude, not my physical health. I was even able to feel grateful for my open incision and ostomy bag, because they were saving my life. I was grateful for the painful and messy procedures, because they were leading to recovery—and on how these treatments would not have been available had this happened when I was a child. And I learned many precious lessons about myself, God's goodness, and the goodness of my family and friends that I still hold dear today.

Now, several years later, I know too that I have been able to show up in a much more sensitive manner for my patients with severe bowel diseases, because I have walked in their shoes. This makes me very glad.

CHAPTER 10

What About Other Treatments?

You might be wondering what else you can do to address your illness anxiety. The previous chapters have given you a quick course in the best strategies for self-help that science has shown are most likely to work for most people. If you try these strategies and follow through with them, there's a good chance that you'll experience success in overcoming your illness anxiety.

But what if these strategies are not enough? What if you're the kind of person who does best when you have some accountability with another person? What if your anxiety is severe enough that the exercises in this book feel too challenging for you to attempt on your own? Or, what if you prefer to use alternative and complementary approaches to well-being, such as acupuncture, massage, essential oils, or Ayurveda?

This chapter will give you suggestions and guidelines about how to find a therapist, medication, or alternative treatment that might help you on your journey to recovery and joy.

First, let me tell you about Joan.

Joan's Story

Joan loved reading self-help books and taking charge of her health care. She ate organic foods as much as possible and enjoyed taking a regular yoga class. She was a trim, athletic person who enjoyed biking, hiking, and swimming. She took vitamins and used lavender and bitter orange oils in a diffuser to help calm her anxiety. She ate a mostly vegetarian diet to improve her health.

Joan also suffered from illness anxiety and felt really frustrated that her own attempts to calm and prevent her anxiety had been unsuccessful. She told me, "I believe that the body can heal itself and I prefer to take a natural approach to healing my body and mind. I'm just so frustrated that I cannot get on top of my fears about getting sick, especially since I know that I'm doing all of the right things that mean I should live a long and healthy life. I want to address my whole person. I'm the healthiest person I know. Why can't I get over my anxiety?"

You might identify with Joan's efforts to live a well-rounded healthy life, especially since you might be the same kind of person, since you're reading this book. You might also feel puzzled about why your efforts to get past your fear don't seem to be working well enough.

Self-help strategies are the best place to start, especially if you know that you're the kind of person who enjoys charting your own path and taking a go at independently making progress before you ask for the help of a professional. This book has been written for you!

When I think about how I prioritize various treatments to recommend to the people I see, I use the following approach that I learned in graduate school. Use well-researched, most-likely-to-succeed treatments first. Always use the treatments that have the least side effects and are least invasive first. Try less expensive treatments first when they are well-researched. If these fail, or give incomplete results, then look to treatments that are considered non-traditional, but have a good body of research. If these fail, then go to any treatments that a group of people seem to find effective. If these fail, then try everything else.

Taking this approach will make it easier for you to embark on a thorough, cost-effective, and efficient approach to your recovery. The first area I will review is things you can do yourself, besides reading this book.

Things You Can Do Yourself

The five areas that you can work on yourself are having an optimal diet, optimal exercise, optimal sleep, learning to meditate, and using evidence-based self-help media, such as this book.

When you eat a diet that is mostly vegetables and fruits, avoid refined or processed foods, stick to organic foods and avoid alcohol, soda/cola drinks, and sweets, you decrease your anxiety, depression, and markers of inflammation (Link, Hassaini, and Jacobson 2005, Null, Penesi, and Feldman 2016). When you exercise regularly for an average of fifty minutes every day, five to six days a week, you reap the benefit of improved physical *and* mental health (Saeed, Cunningham, and Bloch 2019). Additionally, if you keep a regular sleep/wake schedule and get eight to nine hours of sleep each night, then you'll give yourself a mental health advantage (Chattu et al. 2018).

Lastly, if you learn to meditate or engage in daily meditative prayer, you'll give yourself a mental health advantage against anxiety (Lorenc et al. 2018, Vandampfort et al. 2021). If you check the references cited in the back of this book, or read some of New Harbinger's publications about sleep, exercise, diet, and meditation, you can find helpful strategies for improving these areas in your life.

Seeking Professional Help

When self-help approaches—such as reading self-help books, a good exercise routine, maintaining excellent nutrition, excellent sleep, and trying mindful meditation—don't work, I suggest that you seek professional help. Self-help strategies work well for many people whose symptoms are in the mild to moderate range, but often are not enough when your symptoms are moderate to severe.

If you're wise, then you realize that getting the help of an expert can be priceless, because it gives you the opportunity to have an objective expert figure out how better to help you reduce your symptoms and live with joy and purpose. They are also likely to know about the latest information on new or better treatments, and how best to evaluate whether or not it's worth your time and money to try some of them.

Professional help is also an excellent choice when you know you're the kind of person who does better when there's someone who can hold you accountable. If you need accountability, then it's wise to find someone who can help you set and achieve your goals for good mental health.

Finding a Therapist

Cognitive behavioral psychotherapy is the first, best choice for getting the help you need.

When you're looking for a mental health care provider, there are several questions to ask, in addition to how much treatment might cost. Here is a list of helpful questions.

- What is your treatment approach for illness anxiety?
- What is your experience working with people who have illness anxiety?
- What do you think are the most important skills for me to learn in therapy?
- What do you do if I have difficulty following through with my home practice? Have difficulty stopping reassurance-seeking? Need help getting to a medical visit or procedure? Will you be willing to assist me?
- Are you willing to talk with my health care team and help them better understand my illness anxiety? How often?
- Can you work with me through telehealth if I cannot make it to your office?

If you're working with a therapist who is well-versed in using exposure-based treatment for illness anxiety, they will be willing to leave their office and help you practice in the situations that make you anxious, including at your doctor's office or medical facilities. They are also trained to help you do exposure-based therapies using telehealth. For example, I coach some people through their earbuds, while they hold the video camera on their phone facing out, so I can see and hear what they are doing in an anxiety-provoking exposure practice. In this way, I can live-coach someone through their exposure practice, so they have a better chance of successfully completing it. Many therapists who don't use exposure-based therapies will know of therapists who do. Often, they can help you find someone nearby who can assist you.

Additionally, you should feel safe, comfortable, and validated by your therapist, even when they give you feedback about the things you need to change in order to get better. You should feel like your therapist is a combination of a teacher, mentor, coach, and cheerleader when it comes to your mental health.

If you don't feel comfortable working with a particular therapist, be willing to look for someone else. As a therapist, I know that you might not like working with me, because my personality or even my laugh might not fit you. My colleagues and I never take offense when someone desires a better fit for their therapist. We just want you to get better!

Also, I urge you not to worry if your therapist is young or newly graduated. The more important qualification is your therapist's training. If they have had training in exposure-based therapies for illness anxiety, they will be more effective than a seasoned therapist who lacks formal training in exposure-based treatment for anxiety.

If you cannot find a therapist trained in cognitive behavioral therapies (CBT) that are exposure-based, then you might consider looking for one trained in EMDR (Eye Movement and Desensitization and Reprocessing Therapy). EMDR has a good body of evidence for its effectiveness in treating anxiety disorders, especially post-traumatic stress disorder and possibly panic attacks (Yunitri et al. 2020). Studies on the effectiveness shows that EMDR is no better than cognitive behavioral therapies that use exposure, so if you cannot find a cognitive behavioral therapist, then you might look for an EMDR therapist.

ACT (Acceptance and Commitment Therapy) has been shown to be more effective than talk therapy, but slightly less effective than exposure-based therapies (A-Tjak et al. 2015). ACT might be a good choice if you cannot find a CBT- or EMDR-trained therapist.

I should also mention that just talking to your therapist about your anxiety and what it means is unlikely to help you recover. If all you do is talk and listen during your therapy session, without practicing the skills mentioned in this book, then you're at high risk of staying stuck.

I strongly encourage you to find a professional who knows how to teach you how to face, accept, and overcome your anxiety by actually doing it. Many of the people I see in my office have gone to other talk therapists for years without any positive change in their life, except they better understand why they feel anxious. They are surprised when they begin experiencing improvement as soon as they face their feared thoughts and situations.

Please don't wait to become your better self because you think you need to get to the bottom of your anxiety. Trust me, you can get better whether or not you understand the reasons for your anxiety. This is because the maintaining causes of your anxiety (your avoidance and reassurance-seeking) have nothing to do with the initial cause of your anxiety (genetics, life experiences, lifestyle, avoidance of anxiety, and negative role modeling by others).

Medication

If you're looking for medication, you'll need to find someone who is eligible to prescribe medication, such as a physician, psychiatrist, nurse practitioner, or other prescribing professional. Typically, those who prescribe medications will focus on finding the right medicines to help decrease your anxiety, and only rarely will also provide therapy. This means that you'll likely have to go to two separate professionals if you're both seeking therapy and medication.

Prescribers of medication will want to know about any supplements or vitamins you take, in addition to learning about any other medications or health conditions you have, so make sure to have a ready list of nonprescription pills, powders, or drinks you take on a regular basis.

Lastly, you should know that medications are useful for lowering your anxiety approximately 30–40 percent. If your anxiety is severe, this can make the difference between feeling too overwhelmed to do the type of exercises described in this book and being able to dive into treatment.

Complementary Therapies

There is research that supports alternative and complementary therapies for the treatment of anxiety. Acupuncture, Ayurveda, tai chi, and qigong have all been shown to be helpful for anxiety, although in some cases they may work more slowly, require continuing treatment or practice, or provide significantly smaller levels of improvement than the interventions described in Chapters 1 through 9. (For a review of studies of acupuncture, see Li et al. 2019, Murthy et al. 2010.) You should be sure to ask questions of your alternative therapies treatment provider, to make sure you find someone who has experience treating illness anxiety. Here are some specific questions to ask.

- What is your treatment approach for illness anxiety?
- What is your experience working with people who have illness anxiety?
- What do I need to do to make this treatment work?
- What do you do if I have difficulty following through with my home practice or taking the herbs or supplements you prescribe?
- Are you willing to talk with my health care team and help them better understand what you recommend for my treatment?
- Can you work with me through telehealth if I cannot make it to your office?
- How long should it take for me to see results from this type of treatment?
- What do you do if I don't experience results?

Functional Medicine

You might also consult a functional medicine doctor. This is a relatively new field of medicine that combines both traditional Western medical treatments and alternative and complementary treatments. Your functional medicine treatment provider will be a physician who also has specialized training in areas such as nutrition, the gut-brain relationship for neurotransmitters, systemic imbalances, and metabolic imbalances that are often associated with chronic conditions such as autoimmune diseases, food sensitivities, and conditions that have not responded well to traditional medical interventions.

A functional medicine doctor will likely want to assess the quality of your microbiome, the bacteria, fungi, and viruses that populate your gut and body. They might also look at deficiencies in how you absorb nutrients and trace minerals. They may prescribe both traditional and nontraditional medications that consist of supplements, prebiotics, and/or probiotics. They likely will examine your diet and make recommendations about changes in eating habits, and may prescribe fasting.

Functional medicine practitioners may use Ayurvedic techniques and recommend acupuncture. Working with a functional medicine doctor or nurse practitioner will require your willingness to be patient and persistent in making healthy lifestyle changes. Their goal will be to promote your body's own healing abilities and to attain healthy normal metabolic functioning that promotes recovery from anxiety.

Other Treatment Methods

There are other approaches that are easy to find but have not yet been proven by high-quality research. I would caution you to consider these interventions as something to try *in addition to* proven interventions, rather than to solely rely upon them for the mainstay of your recovery. You should follow the same guidelines and ask the same questions of practitioners as listed previously.

The majority of evidence used by practitioners of these types of therapies is personal testimony. Your practitioner, or someone close to your practitioner, experienced a reduction in their anxiety because of this treatment, and this then became the proof of its success.

This, of course, doesn't mean that the same will happen for you, even though it may be very encouraging to hear someone's testimony of anxiety reduction after wearing healing crystals, using essential oils, or using a healing ceremony. Therefore, I recommend that you first try the interventions listed above. Be cautious about investing a lot of money or time into interventions that lack a strong record of research-proven success.

If nothing has worked, after making a genuine effort with skilled therapists and interventions, then I would recommend diving into alternative interventions with gusto. Not every treatment works for every person the same way. Our science of intervention is not perfect. I would rather have you avoid settling for misery and instead make it your mission to recover fully from your illness anxiety. I just suggest first trying what is most likely to succeed.

I also want to respect your religious, tribal, or cultural heritage, when it comes to your healing. The context of your life matters. My work in developing countries has shown that incorporating traditional and spiritual healing practices can be very helpful. Just as my Buddhist colleagues would call upon Buddhist priests to perform pujas to assist in someone's mental health recovery, I draw upon my church's ancient tradition of healing prayer. I would feel spiritually remiss were I not to pray for my clients, nor seek the prayer of others for my own mental and physical health.

You might be interested in turning to reiki (a form of energy healing) or other energy-based therapies, healing crystals or oils, or special healing ceremonies based upon tribal, spiritual, or ancient practices. Many of these interventions are currently popular and easy to locate. You may know of other alternative interventions that pique your curiosity.

Just keep in mind the idea of proceeding with caution, even though others might have exciting testimonies about the healing they obtained from these interventions. You should trust your own experience and be willing to honestly keep track of your symptoms, so you can tell whether or not an alternative intervention is working well for you. Weigh the cost in time, money, and effort against the benefit in reduced anxiety, reduced reassurance-seeking, and reduced avoidance.

Confidence in Your Recovery

Two problems can make it difficult for you to determine whether or not a treatment is working. This is something that no one talks about and it's important.

The first problem is one of well-intended misperception. Most health care providers tend to assume that their skills are improving over time, and that their clinical outcomes with patients are constantly improving (Boswell et al. 2013, Persons et al. 2016). The problem is that they assume that things are going well with the patient even when they are not! This happens because it feels awkward for the patient to tell their health care provider that they are failing.

Think about what you usually do if you receive a haircut that looks awful or if your meal tastes less than delicious at a restaurant. If you're like most people, you just stay quiet, say everything is fine, and then avoid that restaurant or hair salon. The other problem is, if you're like most people, you have a difficult time telling your doctor or therapist that things are not going well, especially if the person is friendly, treats you well, and tells you that you're making progress.

Many therapists mistake having good rapport with a patient as being a sign of progress, as opposed to carefully inquiring about all the ways that your symptoms increase or decrease in between sessions. They also tend to mistake a decrease of anxiety in their office as a sign of success. While this might be encouraging, it's not as significant as what happens when you're not at your doctor's or therapist's office. The gold standard for treatment is measurable improvement between sessions, as opposed to what happens in the session. Let me give you an example.

Lucas's Story

Lucas got really good at doing imaginal exposure about dying and could visit cemeteries and hospital emergency rooms with his therapist after five weeks of exposure practice. This was a big accomplishment, because he had been avoiding funerals, funeral homes, and cemeteries before this, as he didn't want to think about dying. He also used to avoid any thoughts about dying.

The difficulty, however, was that he was unable to do the same practice on his own. He felt safe doing these exposure practices with his therapist, because he assumed that the therapist would help him if his anxiety got uncontrollable. He had been able to stop reassurance-seeking in between sessions, but was afraid to do any independent exposure practice.

Had his therapist underestimated the value of his in-session willingness to practice difficult things, she would have missed a very important target that needed addressing: Lucas's belief that he could not do any exposure to scary thoughts or situations on his own.

Tracking Your Symptoms

So, the best way to keep yourself on the track to recovery is to measure what is happening before, during, and after treatment. If your treatment is working, you should be decreasing reassurance-seeking, increasing your willingness to face anxiety-provoking situations, decreasing the severity and duration of your anxiety, and decreasing avoidance, worry, and panic attacks. That's it. That is recovery.

Toward that end, I suggest you download the anxiety symptom diary, to help you keep track of your results: www.newharbinger.com/49043. Be sure to track your symptoms prior to starting a treatment, and then to keep tracking your symptoms until you either improve or you determine that your treatment is not working well enough to be worth the cost, time, or effort. This way you can be confident that you're not caught up in someone else's enthusiasm or accidental pressure to agree that you're improving.

Even better, show the symptom diary to your treatment provider. If they are interested in your recovery, they will be glad that you're taking the time to measure your results. They will find your tracking sheets to be helpful for determining what they need to do to best help you recover.

In Conclusion

I hope that you're willing to try the steps described in this book. Your journey to recovery is guaranteed when you take these steps to overcome your illness anxiety. There's no need for you to continue to worry and suffer because you fear for your own health or for someone else's. Your good mental health is precious and worth your effort to secure it.

Your real dilemma is not whether or not you have, or will get, a terrible illness. It's how you'll live well in the life that you have been given. Even if you have to deal with a severe or terminal condition, you know that worry about illness and dying only detracts from the quality of your life. Learning to boldly face the thoughts, sensations, and situations you fear will give you confidence and peace of mind about your life at any age or stage.

Gaining the confidence that comes from learning to live with and overcome anxiety about illness and dying is priceless. It makes it much easier to accept and endure the very human experience of illness, aging, and dying. It also makes room for the blessing of gratitude that gives deep meaning, purpose, and substance to your existence.

My great hope is that you join me and others like you on this courageous and beautiful journey of living well.

Acknowledgments

I would like to thank my husband, Dan, for his dedication to our shared dream of preventing, healing, and overcoming suffering in body, mind, and soul. Thank you to my editors at New Harbinger, Ryan Buresh and Jennifer Holder, for their wise feedback that improved the book and made writing it a pleasure. Thank you too to all of my patients who have had the courage to face their fears. You remind me again and again of the incredible courage, resilience, and mental wellness that is possible for us all, no matter our circumstance.

Resources

Finding Providers Who Work with Illness Anxiety

The Academy of Cognitive Therapy

https://www.academyofct.org

Lists therapists and psychiatrists who have special certification in providing evidence-based therapies, many of whom are trained in treating anxiety-related disorders. Listings are also international.

Academy of Integrative Health and Medicine

https://www.aihm.org

Lists licensed and trained medical specialists who practice holistic medicine, such as acupuncture, nutrition, and herbal medicine, along with traditional medicine. They have international listings of members.

Acufinder.com

Provides international listings for providers of acupuncture.

American Massage Therapy Association

https://www.amta.org

Lists licensed providers who maintain the highest standards of care and training in evidence-based methods of massage, reiki, cupping, and other body therapies.

American Society of Acupuncturists

https://www.asa.org

Lists providers who are trained in the use of acupuncture for a wide variety of conditions, including anxiety-related disorders.

Anxiety and Depression Association of America

https://findatherapist.adaa.org

Lists mental health professionals who are familiar with, have expertise in, and enjoy working with people who have anxiety-related disorders, such as illness anxiety. Their website also lists both telehealth and in-person providers of mental health services. Listings are also international.

Association of Behavioral and Cognitive Therapies

https://www.abct.org

Lists mental health professionals who are trained in evidence-based treatments and who specialize in anxiety-related disorders, such as illness anxiety. Listings are also international.

International Association of Reiki Providers

https://www.iarp

Lists providers of reiki.

International Obsessive Compulsive Foundation

https://www.iocdf.org

Lists providers in evidence-based care who are familiar with treatment of illness anxiety. Listings are also international.

Note: Many holistic providers and massage therapists will know of other skilled providers in integrative and complementary therapies that might not be listed in the organizations mentioned above. Just be willing to ask.

References

Algoe, S., S. Gable, and N. Maisel. 2010. "It's the Little Things: Everyday Gratitude as a Booster Shot for Romantic Relationships." *Personal Relationships* 10: 1475-6811.

Allen, S. "The Science of Gratitude." White Paper from the Greater Good Science Center, The John Templeton Foundation, Berkeley, CA. https://ggsc.berkeley.edu/images/uploads/GGSC-JTF_White_Paper-Gratitude-FINAL.pdf?_ga=2.149219826.578176996.1612827107-293062944.1597183668.

American Psychiatric Association. 2013. *Diagnostic and Statistical Manual of Mental Disorders* fifth edition. Washington, D.C.: American Psychiatric Publishing, Inc.

American Psychological Association (APA). "Growing up Grateful Gives Teens Multiple Mental Health Benefits." *ScienceDaily*. 6: August 2012.

A-Tjak, J.G., M.L. Davis, N. Morina, M.B. Powers, J.A. Smits, and P.M. Emmelkamp. 2015. "A Meta-Analysis of the Efficacy of Acceptance and Commitment Therapy for Clinically Relevant Mental and Physical Health Problems." *Psychotherapy and Psychosomatics* 84(1): 30-6.

Amuta, A., R. Miku, W. Jacobs, and A. Ejembi. 2018. "Influence of Cancer Worry on Four Cancer Related Health Protective Behaviors among a Nationally Representative Sample: Implications for Health Promotion Efforts." *Journal of Cancer Education* 33: 1002-1010.

Avallone, K.M., and A.C. McLeish. 2015. "Anxiety Sensitivity as a Mediator of the Association between Asthma and Smoking." *Journal of Asthma* 52(5): 498-504.

Babic, R., M. Babic, P. Rastovic, M. Culin, J. Simic, K. Mandic, and K. Pavlovic. 2020. "Resilience in Health and Illness." *Psychiatry Danub* suppl. 2: 226-232.

Boswell, J.F., D.R. Kraus, S.D. Miller, and M.J. Lambert. 2013. "Implementing Routine Outcome Monitoring in Clinical Practice: Benefits, Challenges, and Solutions." *Psychotherapy Research* published online: 6-19.

Busscher, B., P. Spinhoven, L.J. van Gerwen, and E.J. de Geus. 2013. "Anxiety Sensitivity Moderates the Relationship of Changes in Physiological Arousal with Flight Anxiety during in Vivo Exposure Therapy." *Behavior Research and Therapy* 51(2): 98-105.

Chattu, V.K., M.D. Manzar, S. Kumary, D. Burman, D.W. Spence, and S.R. Pandi-Perumal. 2018. "The Global Problem of Insufficient Sleep and Its Serious Public Health Implications." *Healthcare* (Basel) Dec 20, 2018; 7(1): 1.

Craske, M., M. Treanor, C. Conway, T. Zbozinek, and B. Vervliet. 2014. "Maximizing Exposure Therapy: An Inhibitory Learning Approach." *Behavior Research and Therapy* 58: 10-23.

Davidhizar, R. 1994. "The Pursuit of Illness for Secondary Gain." *Health Care Supervision* 1: 10-5.

Dugas, M.J., P. Gosselin, and R. Ladouceur. 2001. "Intolerance of Uncertainty and Worry: Investigating Specificity in a Nonclinical Sample." *Cognitive Therapy and Research* 25(5): 551-558.

Emmons, R.A., and M.E. McCullough. 2003. "Counting Blessings versus Burdens: An Experimental Investigation of Gratitude and Subjective Well-Being in Daily Life." *Journal of Personality and Social Psychology* 84(2): 377–389.

Fergus, T.A. 2016. "Anxiety Sensitivity and Intolerance of Uncertainty as Potential Risk Factors for Cyberchondria: A Replication and Extension Examining Dimensions of Each Construct." *Journal of Anxiety Disorders* 184: 305-309.

Ferrer R., D. Portnoy, and W. Klein. 2013. "Worry and Risk Perceptions as Independent and Interacting Predictors of Health Protective Behaviors." *Journal of Health Communication* 18: 397-409.

Goyal, M., S. Singh, E. Sibinga, N. Gould, A. Rowland-Seymour, R. Sharma, Z. Berger, D. Sleicher, D. Maron, H. Shihab, P. Ranasinghe, S. Linn, S. Saha, E. Bass, and J. Haythornthwaite. 2014. "Meditation Programs for Psychological Stress and Well-Being: A Systematic Review and Meta-Analysis." *Journal of the American Medical Association: Internal Medicine* 174: 357-68.

Jacoby, R., and J. Abramowitz. 2016. "Inhibitory Learning Approaches to Exposure Therapy: A Critical Review and Translation to Obsessive-Compulsive Disorder." *Clinical Psychology Review* 49: 28-40.

Kabat-Zinn, J. (2005) *Wherever You Go, There You Are: Mindfulness Meditation in Everyday Life*. New York: Hachette Books.

Krause, N., R.A. Emmons, G. Ironson, and P.C. Hill. 2017. "General Feelings of Gratitude, Gratitude to God, and Hemoglobin A1c: Exploring Variations by Gender." *The Journal of Positive Psychology* 12(6): 639–650.

Kreitzer, M.J., S. Telke, L. Hanson, B. Leininger, and R. Evans. 2019. "Outcomes of a Gratitude Practice in an Online Community of Caring." *Journal of Alternative and Complementary Medicine* 25(4): 385-391.

Link, L.B., N.S. Hussaini, and J.S. Jacobson, 2008. "Change in Quality of Life and Immune Markers after a Stay at a Raw Vegan Institute: A Pilot Study." *Complementary Therapies in Medicine* Jun 16(3): 124-30.

Lorenc, A., G. Feder, H. MacPherson, P. Little, S.W. Mercer, and D. Sharp. 2018. "Scoping Review of Systematic Reviews of Complementary Medicine for Musculoskeletal and Mental Health Conditions." *BMJ Open Science* Oct 15, 2018; 8(10): e020222.

McGonigal, K. 2015. *The Upside of Stress: Why Stress Is Good for You, and How to Get Good at It*. New York: Penguin Random House.

McGregor, N., J. Dimatelis, P. Van Zyl, S. Hemmings, C. Kinnear, V. Russell, D. Stein, and C. Lochner. 2018. "A Translational Approach to the Genetics of Anxiety Disorders." *Behavior Brain Research* 341: 91-97.

McLeish A.C, C.M. Luberto, and E.M. O'Bryan. "Anxiety Sensitivity and Reactivity to Asthma-Like Sensations Among Young Adults with Asthma." *Behavior Modification* 40 (1-2): 164-77.

Millstein, R. A., C.M. Celano, E.E. Beale, S.R. Beach, L. Suarez, A.M. Belcher, and J.C. Huffman. 2016. "The Effects of Optimism and Gratitude on Adherence, Functioning and Mental Health Following an Acute Coronary Syndrome." *General Hospital Psychiatry* 43: 17–22.

Persons, J.B. 2007. "Psychotherapists Collect Data during Routine Clinical Work That Can Contribute to Knowledge about Mechanisms of Change in Psychotherapy." *Clinical Psychology: Science and Practice* 14(3): 244-246.

Persons, J.B., P. Koerner, Eidelman, C. Thomas, and H. Liu. 2016. "Increasing Psychotherapists' Adoption and Implementation of the Evidence-Based Practice of Progress Monitoring." *Behavior Research and Therapy* January (76): 24-31.

Ng, M.-Y., and W.-S. Wong. (2013). "The Differential Effects of Gratitude and Sleep on Psychological Distress in Patients with Chronic Pain." *Journal of Health Psychology* 18(2): 263-271.

Null, G., L. Pennesi, and M. Feldman. 2017. "Nutrition and Lifestyle Intervention on Mood and Neurological Disorders." *Journal of Evidence-Based Complementary and Alternative Medicine* Jan 22 (1): 68-74.

Oser M., A. Khan, M. Kolodziej, G. Gruner, A.J. Barsky, and L. Epstein. 2019. "Mindfulness and Interoceptive Exposure Therapy for Anxiety Sensitivity in Atrial Fibrillation: A Pilot Study." *Behavior Modification* 24: 145445519877619.

Parker, Z., G. Waller, P. Gonzalez Salas Duhne, and J. Dawson. 2018. "The Role of Exposure in Treatment of Anxiety Disorders: A Meta-Analysis." *International Journal of Psychology and Psychological Therapy* 18: 111-141.

Pitts, M.J. 2018. "The Language and Social Psychology of Savoring: Advancing the Communication Savoring Model." *Journal of Language and Social Psychology* 38: 237.

Randolph, S. 2017. "The Power of Gratitude." *Workplace Health Safety* 65: 144.

Reiss, S., R. Peterson, D. Gursky, and R. McNally. (1986). "Anxiety Sensitivity, Anxiety Frequency, and the Prediction of Fearfulness." *Behavior Research and Therapy* 24: 1-8.

Sabourin B.C., S.H. Stewart, M.C. Watt, and O.E. Krigolson. 2015. "Running as Interoceptive Exposure for Decreasing Anxiety Sensitivity: Replication and Extension." *Cognitive Behavioral Therapy* 44 (4): 264-74.

Saeed, S.A., K. Cunningham, and R.M. Bloch. 2019. "Depression and Anxiety Disorders: Benefits of Exercise, Yoga, and Meditation." *American Family Physician* May 15, 99(10): 620-627.

Scarella, T., R. Boland, and A. Barsky. 2019. "Illness Anxiety Disorder: Psychopathology, Epidemiology, Clinical Characteristics, and Treatment." *Psychosomatic Medicine* 81: 398-407.

Schwartz, B., A. Ward, J. Monterosso, S. Lyubomirsky, K. White, and D. Lehman. (2020). "Maximizing versus Satisficing: Happiness Is a Matter of Choice." *Journal of Personality and Social Psychology* 83: 1178-1197.

Sirois, F. M., and A. M. Wood. 2016. "Gratitude Uniquely Predicts Lower Depression in Chronic Illness Populations: A Longitudinal Study of Inflammatory Bowel Disease and Arthritis." *Health Psychology* 36(2): 122–132.

Smith, M., S., Sherry, S. Chen, D. Saklofske, C. Mushquash, G. Flett, and P. Hewitt. 2018. "The Perniciousness of Perfectionism: A Meta-Analytic Review of the Perfectionism-Suicide Relationship." *Journal of Personality* 86: 522-542.

Tala, A. 2019. "Thanks for Everything: A Review on Gratitude from Neurobiology to Clinic." *Revista Medica de Chile* 147: 755-761.

Tolin, D. 2019. "Inhibitory Learning for Anxiety Disorders." *Cognitive Behavioral Practice* 26: 225-236.

Vancampfort, D., B. Stubbs, T. Van Damme, L. Smith, M. Hallgren, F. Schuch, J. Deenik, S. Rosenbaum, G. Ashdown-Franks, J. Mugisha, and J. Firth. 2021. "The Efficacy of Meditation-Based Mind-Body Interventions for Mental Disorders: A Meta-Review of 17 Meta-Analyses of Randomized Controlled Trials." *Journal of Psychiatric Research* Feb; 134: 181-191.

Ven Murthy, M.R., P.K. Ranjekar, C. Ramassamy, and M. Deshpande. 2010. "Scientific Basis for the Use of Indian Ayurvedic Medicinal Plants in the Treatment of Neurodegenerative Disorders: Ashwagandha." *Central Nervous System Agents in Medicinal Chemistry* Sep 1; 10(3): 238-46.

Watt, M.C., S.H. Stewart, M.J. Lefaivre, and L.S. Uman. 2006. "A Brief Cognitive-Behavioral Approach to Reducing Anxiety Sensitivity Decreases Pain-Related Anxiety." *Cognitive Behavior Therapy* 35(4): 248-56.

Williams, L.A. and M.Y. Bartlett. 2014. "Warm Thanks: Gratitude Expression Facilitates Social Affiliation in New Relationships via Perceived Warmth." *Emotion,* DOI: 10.1037/emo0000017

Wilson, R. 2009. *Don't Panic: Taking Control of Anxiety Attacks,* third edition. New York: Harper Collins.

Yoshimura, S. and K. Berzins. 2017. "Grateful Experiences and Expressions: The Role of Gratitude Expressions in the Link between Gratitude Experiences and Well-Being." *Review of Communication* 17: 106.

Zvolensky, M.J., J.L. Goodie, D.W. McNeil, J.A. Sperry, and J.T. Sorrell, 2001. "Anxiety Sensitivity in the Prediction of Pain-Related Fear and Anxiety in a Heterogeneous Chronic Pain Population." *Behavior Research and Therapy* 39(6): 683-96.

Zvolensky, M.J., L. Garey, T.A. Fergus, M.W. Gallagher, A.G. Viana, J.M. Shepherd, N.A.Mayorga, L.P. Kelley, J.O. Griggs, and N.B. Schmidt. 2018. "Refinement of Anxiety Sensitivity Measurement: The Short Scale Anxiety Sensitivity Index (SSASI)." *Psychiatry Research* 269: 549-557.

Karen Lynn Cassiday, PhD, is owner and clinical director of the Anxiety Treatment Center of Greater Chicago, the upper Midwest's longest-running exposure-based treatment center for anxiety disorders. She has served as president of the Anxiety and Depression Association of America (ADAA); chair of the scientific advisory board of Beyond OCD; and has published numerous articles, a book for parents of anxious children, and numerous scientific publications that advance the understanding of anxiety disorders. She is a popular commentator in the media, radio show host, and TEDx presenter. She is also clinical assistant professor in the department of clinical psychology at Rosalind Franklin University of Medicine and Sciences. She won the prestigious Clinician of Distinction Award from the ADAA, is an ADAA clinical fellow, a founding fellow of the Academy of Cognitive Therapy (ACT), and one of its certified trainers.

Foreword writer **Simon Rego, PsyD**, is a board-certified cognitive behavioral psychologist with more than twenty years of experience. He is chief psychologist, director of psychology training, and director of the cognitive behavioral therapy (CBT) training program at Montefiore Medical Center in New York, NY. He is also associate professor of clinical psychiatry and behavioral sciences at the Albert Einstein College of Medicine.

ABOUT US

Founded by psychologist Matthew McKay and Patrick Fanning, New Harbinger has published books that promote wellness in mind, body, and spirit for more than forty-five years.

Our proven-effective self-help books and pioneering workbooks help readers of all ages and backgrounds make positive lifestyle changes, improve mental health and well-being, and achieve meaningful personal growth. In addition, our spirituality books offer profound guidance for deepening awareness and cultivating healing, self-discovery, and fulfillment.

New Harbinger is proud to be an independent and employee-owned company, publishing books that reflect its core values of integrity, innovation, commitment, sustainability, compassion, and trust. Written by leaders in the field and recommended by therapists worldwide, New Harbinger books are practical, reliable, and provide real tools for real change.

newharbingerpublications

Did you know there are **free tools** you can download for this book?

Free tools are things like **worksheets**, **guided meditation exercises**, and **more** that will help you get the most out of your book.

You can download free tools for this book—whether you bought or borrowed it, in any format, from any source—from the New Harbinger website. All you need is a NewHarbinger.com account. Just use the URL provided in this book to view the free tools that are available for it. Then, click on the "download" button for the free tool you want, and follow the prompts that appear to log in to your NewHarbinger.com account and download the material.

You can also save the free tools for this book to your **Free Tools Library** so you can access them again anytime, just by logging in to your account! Just look for this button on the book's free tools page.

+ Save this to my free tools library

If you need help accessing or downloading free tools, visit **newharbinger.com/faq** or contact us at **customerservice@newharbinger.com.**